Essential Facts in
Cardiovascular Medicine

Essential Facts in Cardiovascular Medicine

BOARD REVIEW AND CLINICAL PEARLS

Yerem Yeghiazarians, MD
Professor of Medicine
Leone-Perkins Family Endowed Chair in Cardiology
UCSF Medical Center
San Francisco, CA

Rutgers University Press Medicine
New Brunswick, Camden, and Newark, New Jersey, and London

Library of Congress Cataloging-in-Publication Data

Names: Yeghiazarians, Yerem, author.
Title: Essential facts in cardiovascular medicine : board review
    and clinical pearls / Yerem Yeghiazarians.
Description: New Brunswick, New Jersey : Rutgers University
    Press, [2017] | Includes bibliographical references and index.
Identifiers: LCCN 2017038604 | ISBN 9780813579689
    (pbk. : alk. paper) | ISBN 9780813592473 (Mobi) | ISBN
    9780813579696 (epub) | ISBN 9780813579702 (Web PDF)
Subjects: | MESH: Cardiovascular Diseases | Handbooks
Classification: LCC RC667 | NLM WG 39 | DDC 616.1—dc23
LC record available at https://lccn.loc.gov/2017038604

A British Cataloging-in-Publication record for this book is
available from the British Library.

Executive Editor: Kel McGowan
Compositor: Westchester Publishing Services

www.rutgersuniversitypress.org

Manufactured in the United States of America

Contents

Abbreviations

AAA	abdominal aortic aneurysm
ACC	American College of Cardiology
ACE	angiotensin-converting enzyme
ACS	acute coronary syndrome
AHA	American Heart Association
ALCAPA	anomalous left coronary artery arising from the pulmonary artery
ANCA	antineutrophil cytoplasmic antibodies
APLS	antiphospholipid antibody syndrome
AR	aortic regurgitation
ARB	angiotensin receptor blocker
ARC	Academic Research Consortium
ARNI	angiotensin receptor-neprilysin inhibitor (valsartan/sacubitril)
ARVD	arrhythmogenic right ventricular dysplasia
AS	aortic stenosis
ASCVD	atherosclerotic cardiovascular disease
ASD	atrial septal defect
AV	aortic valve
AVA	aortic valve area
AVNRT	atrioventricular nodal reentrant tachycardia
AVRT	atrioventricular reentrant tachycardia
BMI	body mass index
BP	blood pressure
BSA	body surface area
CABG	coronary artery bypass grafting
CAD	coronary artery disease
CCA	common carotid artery
CEA	carotid endarterectomy

CHF	congestive heart failure
CMP	cardiomyopathy
CMV	cytomegalovirus
CO	cardiac output
COPD	chronic obstructive pulmonary disease
CPVT	catecholaminergic polymorphic ventricular tachycardia
CRT	cardiac resynchronization therapy
CTA	computed tomography angiography
CTEPH	chronic thromboembolic pulmonary hypertension
CTO	chronic total occlusion
CV	cardiovascular
DBP	diastolic blood pressure
DLCO	diffusing capacity of the lungs for carbon monoxide
DVT	deep vein thrombosis
EBV	Epstein-Barr virus
EF	ejection fraction
EKG	electrocardiogram
ERO	effective regurgitant orifice
FBG	fasting blood glucose
FDA	Food and Drug Administration
FMD	fibromuscular dysplasia
GI	gastrointestinal
HCM	hypertrophic cardiomyopathy
HDL	high-density lipoprotein
HF	heart failure
HFpEF	heart failure preserved ejection fraction
HFrEF	heart failure reduced ejection fraction
HIV	human immunodeficiency virus
HR	heart rate
HTN	hypertension
IABP	intra-aortic balloon pump
ICA	internal carotid artery
ICD	implantable cardioverter defibrillator
IM	intramuscular
IMI	inferior myocardial infarction
IV	intravenous
IVC	inferior vena cava
JVP	jugular venous pressure
LA	left atrium

LAA	left atrial appendage
LAD	left anterior descending artery
LAE	left atrial enlargement
LAFB	left anterior fascicular block
LBBB	left bundle branch block
LCx	left circumflex artery
LDL	low-density lipoprotein
LMWH	low molecular weight heparin
LOE	level of evidence
LPFB	left posterior fascicular block
LV	left ventricular
LVEDD	left ventricular end-diastolic diameter
LVEDP	left ventricular ejection fraction
LVEF	left ventricular ejection fraction
LVESD	left ventricular end-systolic diameter
LVH	left ventricular hypertrophy
MACE	major adverse cardiovascular event
MAP	mean arterial pressure
MI	myocardial infarction
mPAP	mean pulmonary artery pressure
MR	mitral regurgitation
MRI	magnetic resonance imaging
MS	mitral stenosis
MV	mitral valve
MVP	mitral valve prolapse
NO	nitric oxide
NSAID	nonsteroidal anti-inflammatory drug
NSTEMI	non-ST elevation myocardial infarction
NYHA	New York Heart Association
PAD	peripheral artery disease
PAH	pulmonary arterial hypertension
PAP	pulmonary artery pressure
PCI	percutaneous coronary intervention
PDA	patent ductus arteriosus
PE	pulmonary embolism
PFO	patent foramen ovale
PH	pulmonary hypertension
PHT	pressure halftime
PPM	permanent pacemaker
PR	pulmonic regurgitation

PS	pulmonic stenosis
PV	pulmonic valve
PVR	pulmonary vascular resistance
RA	right atrium
RAD	right anterior descending artery
RAE	right atrial enlargement
RAS	renal artery stenosis
RBBB	right bundle branch block
RCA	right coronary artery
RV	right ventricular
RVEDP	right ventricular ejection fraction
RVH	right ventricular hypertrophy
SAVR	surgical aortic valve replacement
SBP	systolic blood pressure
SC	subcutaneous
SLE	systemic lupus erythematosus
STEMI	ST elevation myocardial infarction
SVC	superior vena cava
SVG	saphenous vein graft
SVR	systemic vascular resistance
SVT	supraventricular tachycardia
TAA	thoracic aortic aneurysm
TAPSE	tricuspid annular plane systolic excursion
TAVR	transcatheter aortic valve replacement
RB	tuberculosis
TEE	transesophageal echocardiography
TG	triglyceride
TLR	target lesion revascularization
TOF	tetralogy of Fallot
TR	tricuspid regurgitation
TS	tricuspid stenosis
TTE	transthoracic echocardiography
TV	tricuspid valve
TVI	time-velocity integral
UFH	unfractionated heparin
VSD	ventricular septal defect
VT	ventricular tachycardia
WHO	World Health Organization
WPW	Wolff-Parkinson-White

Preface

WHY THIS BOOK?

Cardiovascular disease has seen rapid advances over the past few decades. Learning and keeping up with this field is becoming increasingly challenging. In a field with increasing demands in CME, updates in practices, and advances in evidence-based care, one does not always have the luxury of perusing the comprehensive and detailed tomes that have traditionally been the standard. This book is meant to fill that need: to provide the key facts of cardiovascular medicine that every trainee and health care provider needs to know and every expert of cardiovascular medicine will enjoy reviewing, in a format that is high yield and easy to navigate. In essence, *Essential Facts in Cardiovascular Medicine* is a distillation of the most important parts of the field of cardiology, and as such, this book is meant to enhance one's cardiovascular knowledge, prepare one for the board examinations, and improve one's clinical practice.

This book covers numerous important topics from the basics of Statistics, to factoids in General Cardiology, Physical Exam, EKG, Congenital Heart Disease, Valvular Heart Disease, Heart Failure/Transplant, Acute Coronary Syndromes, Pericardial Diseases, Electrophysiology, Pharmacology, Pregnancy, Pulmonary Hypertension, Peripheral Vascular Disease, Echocardiography, Interventional Cardiology, Cardiac Tumors, and Formulas.

Essential Facts in Cardiovascular Medicine is a product of many years of my own career as first a student of cardiovascular medicine during medical school, residency, and fellowship training and then as a teacher–chief resident and then an attending. I put this manuscript together from the many notes that I had taken over the years, the books and journals that I have read, the teachings and mentoring that I have received, and the many conferences that I have attended.

When I was studying for my own board recertification, I could not find a book that covered all the important topics of cardiovascular care in a detailed and concise manner. The best and most comprehensive resources are not ideal for this type of quick review, simply because they are so all-encompassing. As such, *Essential Facts in Cardiovascular Medicine* is structured in bullet/factoid format—it is thorough, is to the point, and covers the common topics as well as the less frequent and often forgotten topics! This book assumes that the reader already has a basic background in medicine and cardiology.

Recommendations listed in this book are per the current guidelines and knowledge in the field. With the nature of rapid advances in the field, it should be understood that some of our current practices and guidelines might change in years to come. We will update future editions to reflect these changes as and when they happen.

Yerem Yeghiazarians, MD

Acknowledgments

I would like to thank my wife, Suzie, and my children, Sofia and Leo, for all their love and support in allowing me to not only complete this book but also to dedicate myself to what I love doing professionally—taking care of patients, teaching the next generation of doctors, and conducting scientific research. I also want to thank my mom, dad (who passed away during the writing of this book but he was extremely proud of the accomplishment), and my brother for their continued support. Last but not least, I would like to thank all my teachers, mentors, trainees and patients over the years for making me a better person and a better doctor.

1 Statistics

- Sensitivity: "true positive"; calculate per Figure 1.1: (A)/(A + C)
- Specificity: "true negative"; calculate per Figure 1.1: (D)/(B + D)
- Positive predictive value: calculate per Figure 1.1: (A)/(A + B)
- Negative predictive value: calculate per Figure 1.1: (D)/(C + D)

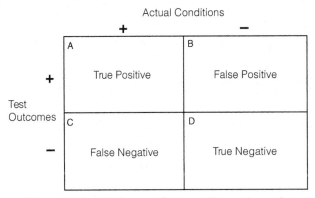

Figure 1.1 Sensitivity, specificity, positive and negative predictive value calculation.

- Type I error (α): reporting a difference when no difference exists ("false positive")
- Type II error (β): reporting no difference when a difference exists ("false negative")

- Power = 1 – type II error (β)
- Likelihood ratio positive (LR+) = sensitivity/(1 – specificity)
- Likelihood ratio negative (LR–) = (1 – sensitivity)/specificity
- Prevalence = actual condition / total population
- Odds ratio = LR+/LR–
- Posttest odds of disease = pretest odds of disease × LR
- Number needed to treat (NNT) = 1/(absolute risk reduction or risk difference)
- Absolute risk reduction (ARR): difference between event rates in the experimental and control groups
- Propensity score matching: method to adjust for observed characteristics of patients randomly assigned differing treatments
- Relative risk (RR): ratio of the probability of an event occurring in an exposed group over a comparison, nonexposed group
- Odds ratio (OR): measure of association between an exposure and an outcome. The OR represents the odds that an outcome will occur given a particular exposure compared to the odds of the outcome occurring in the absence of that exposure.

2 General Cardiology

- Framingham Risk Score includes (Ridker, Buring, Rifai, et al. 2007):
  - Age
  - Sex
  - Total cholesterol
  - High-density lipoprotein (HDL) cholesterol
  - Systolic blood pressure (SBP)
  - Smoking (Wilson, D'Agostino, Levy, et al. 1998)
- Reynolds Risk Score (for healthy patients without diabetes) includes:
  - Age
  - Total cholesterol (mg/dL)
  - HDL cholesterol (mg/dL)
  - SBP (mm Hg)
  - Current smoking (yes or no)
  - Parental history of myocardial infarction (MI) before age 60 years (yes or no)
  - Serum high-sensitivity C-reactive protein (hs-CRP) (mg/L)
- Reynolds Risk Score includes hs-CRP and parenteral history of MI but not body mass index (BMI) or prediabetic status
- Atherosclerotic cardiovascular disease (ASCVD) risk includes age, sex, race, total cholesterol, HDL cholesterol, SBP, blood pressure (BP)–lowering medication use, diabetes status, and smoking status (Goff, Lloyd-Jones, Bennett, et al. 2014)
  - This includes all the Framingham risk factors but also includes race and diabetes
  - It also provides 10-year and lifelong risk

- Incidence of coronary artery disease (CAD) in women has a delayed presentation behind men by about 10 years
- Primary prevention with aspirin is controversial and should be individualized based on risk of bleeding vs potential cardiovascular benefit. In general, assuming patient is not at high bleeding risk, one might consider baby aspirin treatment for patients with a 10-year risk of >10% for cardiovascular (CV) disease, especially with diabetes
- It is controversial but Naproxen might be a better choice over other nonsteroidal anti-inflammatory drugs (NSAIDs) in patients with CV disease but limiting use is strongly preferred
- Sleep Apnea:
  - Central sleep apnea → neural drive to respiratory muscles is abolished
  - Obstructive sleep apnea (OSA) → occlusion of the oropharyngeal airway
  - Apnea-hypopnea Index (AHI) can be used to assess severity of OSA:
    - Mild OSA – AHI ≥ 5 to <15
    - Moderate OSA – AHI ≥ 15 to <30
    - Severe OSA – AHI ≥30
  - OSA contributes to numerous cardiovascular diseases, including:
    - HTN, including resistant HTN
      - AHI 5–15 → odds ratio of HTN 2.0
      - AHI ≥ 15 → odds ratio of HTN 2.9
      - Resistant HTN (difficult to treat requiring 3 drugs at max doses) is associated with OSA in 70–80% of patients
    - Atrial Fibrillation (4 fold higher risk of AF with OSA)
      - Untreated OSA impairs the ability to control AFib
      - Patients with OSA are more likely to have AF recurrences after a cardioversion or catheter ablation
    - Sick sinus syndrome in up to 18% of patients with OSA
    - VT and sudden cardiac death

- Endothelial dysfunction and Coronary artery disease
- Pulmonary HTN
- Heart Failure
- 2–3 fold higher risk of deep vein thrombosis
- 2 fold increased risk of stroke
- 30% higher risk of diabetes with severe OSA
- OSA increases risk of anesthesia and surgery
- Severe OSA associated with increased all-cause mortality and also cardiovascular mortality

HYPERTENSION

Table 2.1 provides a definition for hypertension (HTN).

Table 2.1 Classification of HTN

Normal	<120/80 mm Hg
Pre-HTN	120–139/80–89 mm Hg
Stage 1 HTN	140–159/90–99
Stage 2 HTN	≥160/≥100 mm Hg

Source: James, Oparil, Carter, et al. 2014.

- Risk of cardiovascular disease increases 2-fold for every 20-mm Hg increase in SBP and 10-mm Hg increase in diastolic blood pressure (DBP)
- Around 75% of patients with heart failure have a history of HTN, and HTN increases risk of diastolic heart failure
- Resistant HTN is defined as persistent HTN despite maximal doses of 3 drugs (including a diuretic)
- Causes of HTN: essential >90% of the time and secondary ~10%
- Secondary HTN: younger age; sudden onset; refractory HTN
  - Differential includes:
    - Renal disease
    - Fibromuscular dysplasia (FMD) (more commonly younger female patient)
    - Hyperaldosteronism/Cushing disease
    - Pheochromocytoma

- Aortic coarctation
- Thyroid disease/myxedema
- Sleep apnea
- Oral contraceptive pills
- Steroids
- Licorice
- NSAIDs

- Primary aldosteronism results in ↑serum aldosterone and ↓ plasma renin activity (these are the best screening tests for this condition); also, the serum potassium might be low
- Licorice-induced HTN → licorice inhibits 11-β-OH dehydrogenase, and this results in an increase in cortisol/aldactone level → which causes HTN
- Guidelines in terms of goals of treatment for HTN continue to change. In general, aim for BP of < 140/90 mm Hg; a lower target of < 130/80 mm Hg may be appropriate in some individuals with CAD, previous MI, stroke, or transient ischemic attack (TIA) or CAD risk equivalent but DBP should not be lowered <60 mm Hg.
- Treatment of HTN has many benefits including:
  - Risk of MI decreases by ~20% to 25%
  - Risk of stroke decreases by ~30% to 40%
  - Risk of heart failure decreases by ~40% to 50%
- African American patients respond better to calcium channel blockers and diuretics
- Clonidine can cause sexual dysfunction
- Angiotensinogen (via mechanism of renin) forms angiotensin-converting enzyme (ACE) I, which (via mechanism of ACE) forms ACE II, which leads to:
  - ↑ aldosterone level and ↑ vasopressin
  - Direct vasoconstriction
  - Stimulates oxidase activity and production of free radicals
- With hypertensive emergencies, decrease the mean arterial pressure (MAP) slowly by ~25% within the first couple of hours with intravenous (IV) medications (eg, labetalol, nitroprusside, nicardipine)

DIABETES

- Fasting plasma glucose ≥126 mg/dL
  - 2-hour postglucose load ≥200 mg/dL
  - Diagnosis of diabetes if A1C ≥6.5 or fasting blood sugar is ≥126 mg/dL
  - Goal A1C in diabetic patient with atherosclerosis is <7% (more stringent goal in some patients of <6% if this can be achieved without significant hypoglycemia)
  - Goal for waist circumference <40 inches in men and <35 inches in women
  - Goal for BP <140/90 mm Hg or <130/80 mm Hg if chronic kidney disease or diabetes
  - Risk of cardiovascular death ~15% at 8 years
  - Risk of MI ~15% at 8 years
  - Risk of stroke ~5% at 8 years
  - Diabetic patient with chronic limb ischemia has ~40% chance of gangrene and ~15% chance of amputation
  - For every 1% ↑ in A1C, there is a 14% ↑ in risk of MI; 30% ↑ in all-cause mortality
  - Metformin decreases risk of death and MI but do not use in renal failure
  - ACE inhibitor treatment results in ↓ risk of renal dysfunction but there is no change in mortality
  - Glucagon-like peptide 1 (GLP1) agonist (such as exenatide) decreases cardiovascular events/ mortality
  - Avoid using >2 g/d niacin in a diabetic patient
  - High-intensity statins (with Crestor/atorvastatin) recommended in diabetic patients
- Patients with diabetes, known CAD, or atherosclerotic vascular disease should be treated with high-intensity statins

HYPERLIPIDEMIA

- Dyslipidemia:
  - Primary

- Familial causes (eg, hypercholesterolemia, hyper-triglyceridemia, combined hyperlipidemia, dys-betalipoproteinemia, etc)
  - Secondary
    - Endocrine issues (eg, diabetes, thyroid, or Cushing disease)
    - Renal disease (eg, nephrotic syndrome, increase low-density lipoprotein [LDL] and triglycerides [TGs])
    - Hepatic disease
    - Obesity
    - Alcohol (can increase TGs and HDL)
    - Medications (eg, thiazides can increase LDL and TGs)
- $LDL = TC\text{-}HDL - (TG/5)$ (as long as TGs <400–500 mg/dL)
- Prior to the availability of PCSK-9 inhibitor therapy, LDL apheresis could be considered if LDL is >300 mg/dL or LDL >200 mg/dL on treatment prescription in patients with atherosclerosis
- Daily fat intake—some recommendations:
  - Total cholesterol <300 mg/d
  - Trans fat <1%
  - Saturated fat <7%
  - Sodium <1500 mg/d
- 1% decrease in total cholesterol is associated with ~1% decrease in total mortality and ~1.5% decrease in cardiovascular mortality
- Obesity can lower brain natriuretic peptide (BNP) levels
- Consider bariatric surgery if BMI >40 kg/m^2 or BMI 35 to 39 kg/m^2 with obesity-related complications

Table 2.2 Metabolic syndrome (require 3 for diagnosis)

Waist circumference	>40 in. males; >35 in. females
TG	150
HDL	40 in males; 50 in females
BP	≥130/85 mm Hg in males and females
Fasting blood glucose (FBG)	≥100 in males and females

Source: Alberti, Eckel, Grundy, et al. 2009.

- Familial hypercholesterolemia:
  - Autosomal dominant
  - Tendon xanthomas
- Xanthoma striatum (orange/yellow palm discoloration):
  - Type III hyperlipoproteinemia
  - Familial dysbetalipoproteinemia
- Arcus cornea → can be seen in multiple different lipid disorders
- Tangier disease:
  - Low HDL
  - Apo AI/II catabolized
  - CAD can develop in young patients (40-year-olds)
- Treatment of elevated TGs:
  - TG level of >500 mg/dL can increase risk of pancreatitis
  - Consider treatment with fish oil ± fibrates
  - Improved control of diabetes
  - Weight loss/exercise
- Red yeast rice can cause rhabdomyolysis

STRESS TEST

- Some contraindications for stress testing:
  - Critical aortic stenosis
  - Recent acute MI (within a couple of days)
  - Large pulmonary embolus
  - Uncontrolled hypertension
  - Uncontrolled heart failure
  - Uncontrolled arrhythmias
- Indications for stress testing in a diabetic patient (if ≥1 of the following are present):
  - Typical of atypical symptoms
  - Abnormal electrocardiogram (EKG)
  - Presence of peripheral artery disease (PAD) or carotid disease
  - Age ≥35 years, sedentary lifestyle, and planning on exercise program
- Consider defining coronary anatomy by performing cardiac catheter prior to valve surgery if:
  - Male >35 years old

- - Premenopausal female >35 years old with cardiovascular risk factors
  - Postmenopausal female
- Some other high-risk features on cardiac stress testing include:
  - Large ischemic defect on imaging (>5%)
  - Hypotension with exercise
  - Left ventricular (LV) dilation (≥1.21)
  - >2 segments of abnormal wall motion with low-dose dobutamine stress
- Duke Treadmill Score = Exercise Time − (5 × ST deviation [mm]) − (4 × Angina Index [which is 0, 1, or 2]):
  - If score ≥5 → low risk (0.25% annual cardiovascular mortality)
  - If score −10 to 4 → intermediate risk
  - If score ≤−11 → high risk (5% annual cardiovascular mortality) (Mark, Hlatky, Harrell, et al. 1987)
- If there is left ventricular hypertrophy (LVH) on EKG, use the following criteria for ST changes with stress testing:
  - Positive if >2 mm ST depression
  - Suggestive if 1 to 2 mm ST depression
  - Negative if <1 mm ST depression
- In presence of left bundle branch block (LBBB) or Wolff-Parkinson-White (WPW), perform pharmacologic stress testing
  - ST changes in WPW/pre-excitation EKG pattern are not diagnostic
- Presence of left bundle branch block is associated with reduced survival
- Prior to noncardiac surgery, consider noninvasive stress testing if patient has a functional capacity of <4 metabolic equivalents (METS) and ≥3 risk factors (class IIa)
  - Delay noncardiac surgery in patients with unstable angina, active heart failure, severe valvular disease (eg, aortic stenosis [AS] or mitral stenosis [MS] especially as they do not tolerate volume loads), and/or significant arrhythmias (eg, high-grade aortic valve [AV] block, symptomatic bradycardia, ventricular tachycardia [VT])

- Consider using one of the many available cardiac risk stratification score calculators to assess risk of surgery based on patient risk factors and the type of surgery being performed
- Some contraindications to keep in mind for adenosine pharmacologic testing:
  - Asthma or bronchospastic patients with ongoing wheezing
  - Hypersensitivity to adenosine
  - Greater than first-degree heart block without a pacemaker or sick sinus syndrome
  - SBP <90 mm Hg
  - Use of dipyridamole in the last 24 hours or use of xanthines (aminophylline or caffeine) in the last 12 hours
  - Severe sinus bradycardia (heart rate <40 bpm)
- To reverse side effects of adenosine → treat with aminophylline (125 mg, IV by slow infusion [1 minute]); note that the half-life of adenosine is very short and most effects resolve within a minute after stopping the infusion
- Imaging modalities for assessing myocardial viability include:
  - Magnetic resonance imaging (MRI)
  - Low-dose dobutamine echo
  - Rest and 24-hour thallium study
  - Positron emission tomography-fludeoxyglucose (PET-FDG) study
- Hibernating myocardium:
  - Function reduced
  - Blood flow generally reduced
  - Myocardial energy metabolism reduced
  - Improvement of function with revascularization
- Stunned myocardium:
  - Function reduced
  - Postischemic injury but blood flow restored/normal
  - Myocardial energy metabolism normal
  - Recovery of function

CORONARY COMPUTED TOMOGRAPHY ANGIOGRAPHY

- Coronary calcium
  - Calcium score >100 → >2% risk/year of cardiovascular events over 2 to 5 years
  - Any coronary calcium → associated with a relative risk ratio of ~4 for cardiovascular events over 3 to 5 years
  - Calcium score of >1000 → associated with a relative risk ratio of >10 for cardiovascular events over 3 to 5 years
- Some points to remember for coronary computed tomography angiography (CTA):
  - High negative predictive value → great test to rule out disease
  - Positive predictive value is lower
  - Better quality images if regular heart rhythm with heart rate (HR) 50 to 60 bpm
  - If calcium score is high, CTA is less useful
  - Very useful in assessing graft patency

CLINICALLY IMPORTANT PEARLS

- If a patient presents with hemodynamic compromise, keep the following in mind:
  - Hypoxia
  - Hypovolemia
  - Hypothermia
  - Hyper/hypokalemia
  - Tension pneumothorax
  - Tamponade
  - Toxins
  - Thromboembolic event
- Athletic screening: American Heart Association (AHA) does not recommend routine 12-lead EKG prior to athletic participation but further workup should be considered if there is:
  - Exertional chest pain
  - Unexplained syncope/presyncope

  - Dyspnea/fatigue with exertion
  - Cardiac murmur on exam
  - Hypertension
  - Premature death in the family <50 years old
  - Known cardiac condition in family or cardiac-related disability in a close relative <50 years of age.
  - Physical signs of Marfan syndrome or connective tissue disease
- Canadian Classification Score for angina (Campeau 1976):
  - I: angina with strenuous activity only
  - II: angina with slight limitation
  - III: angina with marked limitation (1–2 blocks of walking or 1 flight of stairs)
  - IV: angina to the point that cannot carry on any activity and/or rest pain
- MI definition (Thygesen, Alpert, Jaffe, et al. 2012):
  - Type 1: spontaneous MI related to ischemia due to a primary coronary (eg, plaque erosion and/or rupture)
  - Type 2: MI from ischemia due to either ↑ O_2 demand or ↓ supply (eg, spasm, embolism, anemia, arrhythmias, hypertension)
  - Type 3: sudden unexpected death likely from MI
  - Type 4a: MI associated with percutaneous coronary intervention (PCI)
  - Type 4b: MI associated with stent thrombosis
  - Type 5: MI associated with coronary artery bypass grafting (CABG)
- Stress-induced cardiomyopathy (TakoTsubo cardiomyopathy [CMP]):
  - Associated with emotional stress, trauma, and surgery
  - More common in women
  - More common in patients >60 years old
  - ST changes might mimic ST elevation myocardial infarction (STEMI) and stress-induced CMP is a diagnosis of exclusion
  - Can present with chest pain, shortness of breath, heart failure, and hypotension
  - Majority improve over days to weeks

○ Increased risk of LV thrombus formation with severe akinesis/hypokinesis of the LV apex in some cases

---

Essential Facts: Amyloid

- Restrictive cardiomyopathy
- Age of presentation ~60 years old
- More commonly male
- May be associated with small skin hemorrhages (around eyes)
- AL primary amyloid (multiorgan; 50% cardiac)
- Low volts on EKG
- Biventricular hypertrophy on echo
- Avoid digoxin
- Diurese for heart failure
- Poor prognosis of <1 year with AL amyloid, ~2 to 3 years with mutation in transthyretin (TTR), and ~5 years with senile form of amyloid
- Isolated left atrium (LA) cardiac amyloid with no other organ involvement may be considered for cardiac transplant combined with stem cell transplant

---

- Conditions that increase risk of arterial thrombosis:
  ○ Antiphospholipid antibody syndrome
  ○ Oral contraceptive pill
  ○ Hyperhomocysteinemia
- Antiphospholipid antibody syndrome:
  ○ Not hereditary
  ○ Can cause valvular heart disease
  ○ Patients with this condition can also get CAD and PAD
  ○ Increased risk for premature bypass graft failure
  ○ Increased risk for recurrent fetal loss
- When to test for a possible hypercoagulable state:
  ○ Idiopathic or recurrent clotting
  ○ First episode of clot at young age (<40 years old)
  ○ Clotting at an unusual region of the body
  ○ +family history of clotting
- Hypercoagulable states to check for include:
  ○ Deficiencies in protein C, protein S, and antithrombin III

- ○ Factor V Leiden
- ○ Prothrombin gene mutation (20210)—also called factor II mutation
- ○ Lupus anticoagulant/antiphospholipid Ab syndrome
- Protein C (not S) deficiency → associated with risk of warfarin necrosis
- Glanzman thrombasthemia:
  - ○ Mutation of Gp IIb/III receptor
  - ○ Increased mucocutaneous bleeding
- Von Willebrand disease → factor VIII deficiency (this is not a disorder of platelets)
- Heparin:
  - ○ Inhibits factor II
  - ○ Prolonged heparin treatment can lead to thrombocytopenia, osteoporosis, and alopecia
  - ○ Can cause hyperkalemia by decreasing aldosterone level
- Heparin-induced thrombocytopenia diagnosis:
  - ○ Use serotonin release assay
  - ○ Platelet factor 4 (PF-4) assay is sensitive but has low specificity
  - ○ Treat for at least ~3 months
  - ○ Acute treatment with IV argatroban
  - ○ Warfarin should not be used in heparin induced thrombocytopenia (HIT) until the platelet count is $\geq 150 \times 10^9$/L due to increased risk of developing warfarin necrosis when platelet count is low
- Protamine is given to reverse the heparin effect. But allergic reactions can occur and care should be taken in the following conditions:
  - ○ If patient has allergy to fish
  - ○ If patient is taking NPH insulin (not as much of an issue with regular insulin)
  - ○ Male patients following vasectomy
- Some risk factors for developing deep vein thrombosis (DVT):
  - ○ Pregnancy
  - ○ Obesity
  - ○ Older age
  - ○ Smoking

- Heart failure
- Prior DVT/pulmonary embolism (PE)
- Malignancy
- Nephrotic syndrome
- Medications (eg, oral contraception pills)

Essential Facts: Pulmonary Embolism

- ~1/3 die at 30 days
- ~1/3 recur at 10 years
- ~1/3 may have postphlebitic syndrome
- For large PE that results in BP <90 mm Hg (for >15 minutes), the 90-day mortality >~50%
- For massive PE with hemodynamic compromise (eg, hypotension with SBP <90 mm Hg, severe hypoxemia, right ventricular (RV) dysfunction), consider lytic therapy (tissue plasminogen activator [TPA] 100 mg over 2 hours or weight-adjusted tenecteplase [TNK])
- Catheter-based intervention or thrombectomy can also be considered if large proximal PE with hemodynamic compromise
- Inferior vena cava (IVC) filter can be considered when anticoagulation is contraindicated

---

- For cancer-related DVT/PE → treat with low molecular weight heparin (LMWH) 3 to 6 months, then can consider switching to warfarin
- Duration of therapy for DVT:
  - Treat with long-term anticoagulation if second DVT event or if cancer/hypercoagulable state is present
  - For first provoked DVT event, treat for 3 to 6 months and reassess
  - For first unprovoked DVT, 3 to 6 months but consider longer term therapy pending on the risk of bleeding vs benefit in a given patient (this is more controversial)

- Upper extremity DVT:
  - Rule out thoracic outlet syndrome and if present, rib resection surgery should be performed
  - ~10% risk of PE (but fatal PE is ~1%)
  - Treat for ~3 months of anticoagulation
  - Recurrence rate ~2.5%
  - If catheter induced, remove the catheter

Essential Facts: Rheumatic Fever

- Risk in untreated strep pharyngitis is about 3%
- Inflammatory reaction after group A streptococcal infection
- Major features:
  - Carditis
  - Polyarthritis
  - Chorea
  - Erythema marginatum
  - Subcutaneous nodules
- Minor features:
  - Arthralgias
  - Fever
  - Elevated erythrocyte sedimentation rate (ESR)/ CRP
  - Prolonged PR interval
  - Treatment with penicillin
  - For patients allergic to penicillin, treat with erythromycin

---

- Some facts to remember about some cardiovascular medications/conditions:
  - Treat pheochromocytoma crisis with IV phentolamine
  - Treat amitriptyline overdose with sodium-containing solution
  - Treat cerebral vasospasm due to subarachnoid hemorrhage with nimodipine (calcium channel blocker)
  - Reverse hirudin action by using prothrombin complex
  - Treat cyanide toxicity with:

- Amyl nitrate
- Sodium nitrite
- Sodium thiosulfate
- Mitochondrial disorder can result in "ragged red fibers" on biopsy
- Marfan syndrome → autosomal dominant

Essential Facts: Osteogenesis Imperfect

- Blue sclera
- Mitral valve prolapse (MVP)
- Aortic regurgitation
- Hearing loss
- Fragile bones

Essential Facts: Pseudoxanthoma Elasticum

- Yellow skin papules
- Retinal angioid streaks
- Valve incompetence
- Possible associated heart block

Essential Facts: Carcinoid

- Symptoms might include flushing, diarrhea ± wheezing
- Tumor releases serotonin
- Half of carcinoid patients will have some cardiac involvement
- Keep in mind that ovarian carcinoid tumor (since the ovarian venous system bypasses the portal circulation) can have cardiac involvement without any liver involvement

(continued)

- Most common valve involvement (>90% of the time) are the right-sided valves that result in fibrous thickening
- Left-sided valve involvement is <10% of the time (especially if right-to-left shunting exists or there are pulmonary carcinoid tumors)
- Diagnosis: 5-Hydroxyindoleacetic acid (5-HIAA) 24-hour urine collection; can consider octreoscan
- Consider treatment with octreotide ± surgery

Essential Facts: Methemoglobinemia
- Hemoglobin able to carry oxygen but unable to release it effectively to tissues
- Inherited vs acquired (more common)
- Some causes for acquired form:
  - Benzocaine anesthetic
  - Benzene
  - Other medications:
    - Dapsone
    - Chloroquine
    - Nitrates
    - Note: Sildenafil does not cause methemoglobinemia
- Symptoms can include blue discoloration of skin, shortness of breath, headache, and fatigue
- Treatment:
  - Methylene blue (1–2 mg/kg 1% solution over 5 minutes)
  - If glucose-6-phosphate dehydrogenase (G6PD) deficiency → treat with ascorbic acid 300 to 1000 mg
  - In some cases, might need to consider exchange transfusion

3 Physical Exam

- $0.7 \times$ (jugular venous pressure [JVP] in cm) = pressure in mm Hg
- Order of valve closure:
  - Left-sided valves close before right-sided valves (assuming normal conduction system)
  - "*Many Things Are Possible*"—order of valve closure is *M*itral, *T*ricuspid, *A*ortic, and *P*ulmonic
- Presystolic accentuation refers to atrial contraction (S4)
- Inspiration → A2 – P2, 40 to 60 ms
- Inspiration with a right bundle branch block (RBBB) → A2 – P2, 60 to 80 ms
- Persistent S2 → RBBB and pulmonary HTN
- Fixed splitting of S2 → atrial septal defect (ASD)
- Paradoxical split of S2 → LBBB/paced; critical aortic stenosis; hypertrophic cardiomyopathy (HCM)
- S3:
  - Can be a normal finding in children and young athletes
  - May be present with LV dysfunction
- S4:
  - Absent in atrial fibrillation
  - Left-sided S4—can be heard in the setting of LVH (eg, due to systemic HTN or aortic stenosis)
  - Right-sided S4—can be heard in the setting of RVH (eg, pulmonary HTN)
  - Acute coronary syndrome/myocardial ischemia
- P2 is diminished or might even be absent in pulmonary stenosis

- Loud P2 is associated with pulmonary HTN; definition of loud S2 is that it is increased in intensity and heard at the apex
- Severe mitral regurgitation (MR) on exam can be associated with:
  - S3
  - Systolic thrill
  - ≥4/6 murmur
  - Diastolic rumble
  - Note → murmur of acute mitral regurgitation is early systolic
  - Murmur of mitral regurgitation due to prolapse of the anterior leaflet is typically best heard at apex with radiation to the axilla
  - Severity of mitral stenosis → the shorter the S2-opening interval, the more severe the MS given the higher left atrial pressure that results in early opening of the mitral valve:
    - Severe → S2-opening snap is <70 ms
    - Moderate → S2-opening snap is 70 to 110 ms
    - Mild → S2-opening snap is >110 ms
- There is no S3 with mitral stenosis; possible S3 when chronic MR
- Severe aortic stenosis on exam can be associated with:
  - Delayed peaking murmur
  - Paradoxical S2
  - Pulsus brevis
  - Pulsus tardus
- Gallavardin murmur:
  - High-frequency musical murmur at the cardiac apex due to aortic stenosis (may sound like MR murmur)
    - Post-premature ventricular contraction (PVC), the Gallavardin murmur gets louder but MR murmur does not change
- Carvallo sign:
  - Murmur of tricuspid regurgitation gets accentuated with inspiration
- Aortic regurgitation:
  - Aortic regurgitation (AR) duration (not intensity) correlates with severity

- o Murmur of acute aortic regurgitation is early diastolic and may not even be audible given the acute rise in the left ventricular ejection fraction (LVEDP)
  - o Austin flint murmur → diastolic rumble due to AR can mimic functional MS
  - o Bisferiens pulse → severe AR
- Some of the peripheral signs in patients with aortic regurgitation:
  - o Corrigan's pulse: Rapid and forceful distension of the arterial pulse with a quick collapse
  - o De Musset's sign: Bobbing of the head with each heartbeat
  - o Muller's sign: Visible pulsations of the uvula
  - o Quincke's sign: Capillary pulsations seen on compression of the nail bed
  - o Traube's sign: Systolic and diastolic sounds heard over the femoral artery ("pistol shots")
  - o Duroziez's sign: Gradual pressure over the femoral artery leads to a systolic and diastolic bruit
  - o Hill's sign: Popliteal systolic blood pressure exceeding brachial systolic blood pressure by 60 mm Hg or greater (most sensitive sign for aortic regurgitation)
  - o Shelly's sign: Pulsation of the cervix
  - o Becker's sign: Visible pulsation of the retinal arterioles
  - o Mayne's sign: A decrease in diastolic blood pressure of 15 mm Hg when the arm is held above the head (very nonspecific)
- Two reasons for mid-systolic closure of the aortic valve: (1) HCM and (2) subaortic stenosis
- Some likely physical exam findings in pulmonary HTN:
  - o Loud P2
  - o Right-sided gallop sound
  - o Right ventricular (RV) heave
  - o Pulmonary flow murmur
  - o Elevated JVP
  - o Edema/ascites/hepatomegaly
- Diastolic murmurs are abnormal. Some possible causes:
  - o Aortic regurgitation (murmur starts at A2—aortic component of S2)

- ○ Pulmonic regurgitation (murmur starts at P2—pulmonic component of S2)
  - ○ Mitral stenosis
  - ○ Tricuspid stenosis
- Continuous murmurs can be heard in:
  - ○ Patent ductus arteriosus (PDA)
  - ○ Venous hum
  - ○ Mammary souffle
  - ○ Bronchial collaterals
  - ○ Arteriovenous connection (pulmonary or coronary atrio-venous [AV] fistula)
  - ○ Ventricular septal defect (VSD) and aortic regurgitation
  - ○ Pulmonary artery branch stenosis
  - ○ Rupture of sinus of Valsalva
  - ○ Coarctation of the aorta
- Platypnea orthodeoxia (desaturation with sitting/standing)—possible causes:
  - ○ Patent foramen ovale (PFO)
  - ○ ASD

Table 3.1 Maneuvers and how they affect murmurs of MR, AS, HCM, and VSD

Maneuver	Physiologic Response	MR	AS	HCM	VSD
Handgrip	↑ afterload	+	−	−	+
Squat	↑ afterload/preload	+	−	−	+
Standing	↓ afterload/preload	−	−	+	− or none
Valsalva	↓ preload	−	−	+	− or none
Post-PVC	↓ afterload/↑ constriction	None	+	+	+ or none
Amyl nitrite	↓ afterload	−	+	+	−

Note: +=murmur louder; −=murmur softer; none=no change in murmur.
Source: Mann, Zipes, Libby, et al. 2015; Murphy, Lloyd 2013.

- ○ AV shunts (pulmonary)
- ○ Hepatopulmonary syndrome
- ○ Osler-Weber-Rendu syndrome
- Pulse pressure after a PVC is decreased in HCM (as opposed to AS)
- Bifid pulse → hypertrophic obstructive cardiomyopathy (HOCM)
- Nonejection click can be heard in:
  - ○ MVP
  - ○ Septal aneurysm (atrial or ventricular)
  - ○ Cardiac tumors
  - ○ Pulmonic or systemic HTN
- VSD can result in pansystolic murmur with or without associated palpable thrill
- Only right-sided sound that decreases with inspiration → ejection click of pulmonary stenosis
- Kussmaul sign:
  - ○ Increase or lack of decrease in the JVP with inspiration
  - ○ Commonly associated with constrictive pericarditis but can also be seen in RV failure/infarct, tricuspid stenosis, or cor pulmonale
- Branham's sign:
  - ○ Slowing of the heart rate after compression of an aortovenous fistula

4 EKG

- Left anterior descending artery (LAD) $-30°$ → differential includes Wolff-Parkinson-White (WPW), inferior myocardial infarction (IMI), LVH, and LBBB
- Right anterior descending artery (RAD) $+90°$ → differential includes WPW, PE, right ventricular hypertrophy (RVH), chronic obstructive pulmonary disease (COPD)/pulmonary disease, and lateral MI
- Left anterior fascicular block (LAFB) axis $-45°$ to $-90°$ and qR in I/aVL and QRS <120 ms
- Left posterior fascicular block (LPFB) axis $+100°$ to $180°$ and rS in I/aVL and QRS <120 ms and qR in III/aVF
- Bazett's formula for QTc → $QT/\sqrt{RR}$
- Fridericia's formula for QTc (use at higher or lower heart rates) → $QTc = QT / \sqrt[3]{RR}$
- Short QTc → <340 ms (due to gain of function of potassium channel disease)
- Long QTc → ≥440 ms (male); ≥460 ms (female)
- Diagnosis of LVH (some criteria to consider):
  - Sokolow criteria:
    - SV1+RV5 or 6 → >35 mm (age >30 years)
    - SV1+RV5 or 6 → >40 mm (age 20–30 years)
    - SV1+RV5 or 6 → >60 mm (age 16–20 years)
  - R in I >14 mm; R in avL >12 mm
  - Cornell criteria:
    - R avL + SV3 ≥28 mm (male) or ≥20 mm (female)
- Diagnosis of RVH:
  - R > S in V1 or R in V1 ≥7 mm
  - Decrease in R/S ratio across the precordium
  - Presence of RAD

- ○ Possible rSr' pattern in V1
- ○ Persistent S-wave in left precordial leads
- Some causes of prominent R-wave in V1:
  - ○ RVH
  - ○ WPW
  - ○ Posterior MI
  - ○ RBBB
  - ○ Dextrocardia
  - ○ Lead misplacement
  - ○ Duchenne muscular dystrophy
  - ○ Normal variant
- Some causes of poor R-wave progression across the precordium:
  - ○ Anteroseptal MI
  - ○ Lung disease/COPD/pneumothorax
  - ○ Lead misplacement
- Right ventricular hypertrophy when RBBB is present → R in V1 ≥15 mm and right axis deviation
- Normal atrial-His bundle (AH) interval <150 ms
- Normal His bundle-ventricle (HV) interval <35 to 55 ms
- Easy way to remember pathologic Q-waves:
  - ○ 25% of the height of the QRS or
  - ○ "One small box wide" and "one small box deep"
- Mobitz 1: Improves with exercise/atropine → due to AV-nodal delay
- Mobitz 2: Worsens with exercise/atropine (associated bundle branch block [BBB]) → due to His-Purkinje disease
- WPW—preexcitation pathway (see Table 4.1):
  - ○ Short PR <0.12 ms
  - ○ QRS >0.10 ms
  - ○ Delta wave
- Atrial septal defect—EKG findings:
  - ○ Primum ASD → LAD, RsR', QRS <0.11 s
  - ○ Secundum ASD → RAD, RsR', QRS <0.11 s
- Osborn wave:
  - ○ Abnormal positive deflection at the junction of the QRS/ST segment
  - ○ Associated with hypothermia (<32°C)
  - ○ Rarely in patients with hypercalcemia, brain injury

Table 4.1 Location of accessory pathways
in Wolff-Parkinson-White (WPW)

	V1	aVF	aVL
Left lateral	+	+	−
Left posterior/septal	+	−	+
Right posterior/septal	−	−	+
Right lateral/anterior	−	+	+

Note: + = EKG vector positive; − = EKG vector
negative.

- Duchenne muscular dystrophy:
  - Can have tall R-waves in V1 and qs in the lateral
    leads (I/AvL/V5-6)
  - Creatine kinase (CK)-MB level does not correlate with
    degree of myocardial disease
  - Posterobasal and posterolateral left ventricular walls
    are most affected
- Some causes of ST elevation:
  - Acute MI
  - Pericarditis
  - Takotsubo/stress cardiomyopathy
  - Coronary spasm
  - Hypertrophic cardiomyopathy
  - Brugada
  - Hyperkalemia
  - Hypothermia
  - Early repolarization/LVH
- Pulmonary emboli (can sometimes result in ST elevation in
  precordial leads V1 to V2 and may or may not be associ-
  ated with tachycardia, possibly S1Q3T3, RAD, RBBB)
- ST elevation in aVR:
  - Left main disease
  - Global ischemia
- Definition of low volts:
  - <5 mm in limb leads
  - <10 mm in precordial leads
- Some causes of low volts:
  - Pericardial effusion

- ○ Lung disease/COPD
- ○ Obesity
- ○ Myxedema
- ○ Amyloid/infiltrative myopathy
- ○ Pleural effusion
- Atrial flutter is 2.5 times more common in men and comprises ~10% of supraventricular tachycardias (SVTs)
- Typical atrial flutter → negative axis in leads II/III/aVF (counterclockwise reentry)
- Ventricular tachycardia (some criteria) (see page 83):
  - ○ Initial R wave in aVR or R or Q wave >40 ms
  - ○ Right super axis
  - ○ Onset of R-wave to S-wave >100 ms
- Junctional reciprocating tachycardia usually has a rate of 100 to 130 bpm; associated with inverted P-waves in the inferior leads and is common in patients with dilated cardiomyopathy.
- Hypocalcemia → can result in QT prolongation
- Hypercalcemia → can result in QT shortening

5 Congenital Heart Disease

- Incidence of congenital heart disease:
  - ~1% of babies born
  - ~5% in offspring of women with congenital heart disease
- Anomalous coronary artery:
  - Incidence <~1%
  - Most common anomaly in adults is an anomalous left circumflex artery (25%) arising from the right sinus of Valsalva
    - On ventriculography, "dot" sign can be noted behind the aorta in the right anterior oblique (RAO) view
  - Some cardiac conditions with association with coronary anomalies include:
    - Tetralogy of Fallot:
      - ~10% cases
      - Most commonly LAD from the right coronary artery (RCA) or right sinus of Valsalva
      - Some cases with single coronary artery
    - Transposition of great arteries
    - Truncus arteriosus
- Anomalous left coronary artery arising from the pulmonary artery (ALCAPA):
  - <0.5% of patients with congenital heart disease
  - Usually an isolated cardiac anomaly
  - RCA is very dominant and supplies the myocardium
  - Usually presents with heart failure in infancy but occasionally can be present in adulthood with LV dysfunction/myocardial ischemia/heart failure
  - Surgical correction when diagnosed is recommended

- Cyanotic congenital cardiac conditions that result in increased pulmonary flow:
  - Transposition of the great arteries
  - Truncus arteriosus
  - Total anomalous pulmonary venous return
- Cyanotic congenital cardiac conditions that result in decreased pulmonary flow:
  - Tetralogy of Fallot
  - Tricuspid atresia
- Most common birth cyanotic deficit is transposition
- Most common childhood cyanotic defect is tetralogy of Fallot
- Hyperviscosity in cyanotic heart disease:
  - May occur when hematocrit is >65%
  - Increased risk of hyperviscosity if iron deficiency is also present as the cells are deformed with iron deficiency
    - Treat iron deficiency
    - Keep hydrated
- Patients with cyanotic heart disease may have lower platelet levels/function and lower levels of coagulation factors (hence abnormal prothrombin time/partial thromboplastin time (PT/PTT) levels)—these increase the risk of bleeding in these patients
- L-transposition:
  - Congenitally corrected transposition
  - Presence of both atrioventricular and ventriculo-arterial discordance
  - Morphologic RV is on the left
    - Deoxygenated blood goes from right atrium (RA) → LV (now on the right side) → pulmonary artery (PA)
    - Oxygenated blood returns to LA → RV (now on the left side) → aorta
  - Frequently (>90% of cases) associated with other cardiac abnormalities:
    - Situs solidus
    - Atrial-ventricular valve discordance
    - Ventriculo-arterial discordance
    - Peri-membranous VSD

- Pulmonary stenosis
- Ebstein's anomaly
- Complete heart block
- AV regurgitation with congestive heart failure
- SVT
- Q-waves inferiorly
- At risk for heart failure given that the RV is now the systemic ventricle
- Treatment options:
  - Anatomic repair for pediatric patients with L-transposition of the great arteries (L-TGA) and associated lesions
  - If isolated L-TGA, either surgical anatomic repair vs very close observation to make sure systemic RV is not enlarging/failing
- D-transposition:
  - More common form of transposition
  - Ventriculo-arterial discordance
  - Morphologic RV is on the right
    - Aorta arises from the RV and the pulmonary artery arises from the LV
    - Deoxygenated blood goes from RA → RV → aorta
    - Oxygenated blood returns to LA → LV → PA
    - As such, there are "parallel" circuits, and this is an "uncorrected" transposition → cyanotic congenital heart lesion
  - If no other associated cardiac abnormalities, this is known as "simple TGA"
  - Associated VSD in ~50% of cases
  - Surgical correction
- PFO:
  - Almost one-third of the general population
  - Presence of PFO increases risk of air embolism in scuba divers
  - Possible increased risk of embolization/stroke if the PFO is larger and there is atrial septal aneurysm
- Secundum ASD:
  - More common in females than in males
  - Patients with secundum ASD can be at risk for atrial flutter and sinus node dysfunction

- In secundum ASD, left atrial enlargement (LAE) is unusual unless the patient is >40 years old ± atrial fibrillation
- If patient is young (<~40 years old) and has no atrial fibrillation but the LA is enlarged, rule out primum ASD
- EKG: RAD, RsR'
- Physical exam: fixed split S2; pulmonic ejection murmur, ± RV heave
- Closing secundum ASD does not prevent atrial fibrillation but early closure does ↓ risk of atrial fibrillation
- If ASD is closed before age 25 years, survival is same as non-ASD patients; however, if ASD closure is delayed until >40 years old, then patient outcomes are worse
- Class I recommendation to close ASD when evidence for right-sided volume/pressure overload (eg, RA and RV enlargement)
- Percutaneous closure usually performed when defect is <4 cm and there are at least ~4-mm rims
- After ASD device closure, within 30 days, ~5% of patients might develop atrial arrhythmias
- If nonsustained ventricular tachycardia (NSVT) is noted after ASD device closure, always think of device migration that is resulting in ventricular arrhythmias

- Primum ASD—some associated lesions to keep in mind:
  - EKG: LAD, RsR'
  - Association with Down syndrome
  - Other possible associations:
    - VSD
    - Pulmonic stenosis (PS)
    - Subaortic stenosis
    - Left superior vena cava (SVC) syndrome
    - Coarctation of the aorta
  - Treatment is surgical closure—not amenable to percutaneous closure

- Sinus venosum ASD can be associated with:
  - Anomalous right upper pulmonary vein
  - Left axis deviation

- o Inversion of P-waves on EKG
- o Defect located posterior to the fossa
- o Treatment is surgical closure—not amenable to percutaneous closure
- Anomalous pulmonary vein:
  - o Should be ruled out if RV volume overload is present and there is no ASD
  - o Can be associated with:
    - Sinus venosus ASD (most commonly)
    - VSD
    - Tetralogy of Fallot
- VSD:
  - o Some subtypes:
    - Perimembranous (also otherwise known as membranous/infracristal)—70% to 80% most common type of VSD
    - Muscular—5% to 20%
    - Supracristal (also otherwise known as subaortic or subpulmonic)—5% to 7%
  - o Large VSD might result in Eisenmenger physiology over time
  - o If VSD defect is small, the murmur is loud
  - o Associated VSD is common with pulmonary stenosis (~two-thirds of cases)
  - o Muscular and membranous defects frequently spontaneously close
    - By age 3 years, ~40% to 45% of these VSDs are spontaneously closed
    - Most others close by age 8 to 10 years
  - o Irrespective of symptoms, supracristal defects should be closed as they can result in AR
  - o If asymptomatic perimembranous or muscular VSDs, can observe and no immediate invasive therapy might be needed, unless it is causing increase in cardiac chamber size, increasing right-sided pressure, causing aortic regurgitation, or patient has had recurrent endocarditis
  - o Complete heart block, even though uncommon, can occur after surgical VSD repair

- Tetralogy of Fallot (TOF):
  - Four key malformations include:
    - Pulmonary stenosis
    - VSD
    - Overriding aorta
    - RVH
  - Most common childhood cyanotic defect is TOF
  - Fetal alcohol syndrome and rubella infection in the mother during pregnancy is associated with TOF
  - ~25% right aortic arch
  - ~10% to 15% associated with secundum ASD
  - ~5% to 10% have anomalous coronary arteries (usually LAD arising from the RCA or from the right sinus of Valsalva)
  - Partial or total anomalous drainage; the pulmonary veins can be seen in association
  - Possible exam findings: Cyanosis; RV lift ± thrill if severe pulmonary obstruction; loud systolic murmur due to the pulmonary stenosis and possibly absent P2
  - CXR: "Boat-shaped" heart with a concave pulmonary arterial segment; possible right aortic arch
  - EKG: If QRS >180 ms, worse prognosis
- After TOF repair, patient might develop problems with the pulmonary valve. Indications for pulmonic valve (PV) intervention include:
  - Symptoms
  - Widening QRS >180 ms
  - QRS prolongation >3.5 ms/y
  - Arrhythmias
  - Enlarging RV with RV end systolic volume (ESV) >85 and RV end diastolic volume (EDV) >170
  - Residual right ventricular outflow tract (RVOT) obstruction with right ventricular systolic pressure (RVSP) ≥ two-thirds systemic pressure and/or residual shunt
- Right aortic arch and cyanosis → think of TOF
- Right-sided aortic arch can be associated with:
  - Dysphagia
  - 25% of the time with TOF

- ○ Associated with other anomalies, including truncus arteriosus, transposition of the great arteries, and pulmonary atresia
- ○ Note that this condition is not associated with an ASD
- Patent ductus arteriosus:
  - ○ Maternal rubella increases risk of PDA
  - ○ More common in females
  - ○ Usually wide pulse pressure is present with a machinery continuous murmur
  - ○ Rarely closes after infancy (as opposed to VSD)
  - ○ Early closure of PDA is recommended
  - ○ If not closed, it can result in volume overload on the left side and LA ± LV enlargement and eventually result in pulmonary HTN if left untreated
- Aortic coarctation:
  - ○ More common in males
  - ○ Location frequently distal to the left subclavian artery
  - ○ Rubella infection in mother can increase risk of coarctation
  - ○ Fetal alcohol syndrome can be associated with coarctation
  - ○ Can be associated with Turner syndrome
  - ○ Rule out associated bicuspid aortic valve
  - ○ Rule out associated cerebral aneurysms
  - ○ HTN in the upper extremities with delayed pulses in the lower extremity
  - ○ Possible +S4 due to longstanding HTN
  - ○ Robust collaterals might form from the upper to lower extremity
  - ○ Aortopathy with cystic medial necrosis
  - ○ Chest x-ray (CXR): "Figure 3 sign" and rib notching
  - ○ Consider treating if the peak gradient is ≥20 mm Hg
    - ▪ Endovascular angioplasty/stenting
    - ▪ Surgical repair
  - ○ Risk of aneurysm formation over time is increased with surgical Dacron patch repair, and this requires follow-up routine imaging
  - ○ Despite repair, patients with coarctation have increased mortality

- - Earlier repair appears to be associated with better survival
  - 30-year survival after repair is ~70%
- Triscuspid atresia:
  - There is no direct communication between the right atrium and ventricle
  - Cyanosis
  - Right atrial enlargement
  - Associated conditions—right to left shunting is required for survival:
    - ASD
    - VSD
    - Right ventricular hypoplasia
    - Pulmonary outflow obstruction
  - EKG: Tall P-waves, left axis deviation, LVH (and loss of RV forces)
  - Treatment:
    - Initially support with pulmonary vasodilators (eg, prostaglandin) and then surgical repair (Fontan procedure)
- Ebstein's anomaly:
  - Maternal lithium exposure is associated with Ebstein's anomaly
  - Rubella infection in mother is not associated with Ebstein's anomaly
  - Septal and posterior leaflets are displaced in the right ventricle; the anterior leaflet arises from the normal position on the tricuspid valve
  - Other associated cardiac shunts:
    - PFO/ASD in ~50%
    - Association with VSD
  - Exam:
    - Can be associated with tricuspid regurgitation with holosystolic murmur, which is accentuated with inspiration
    - Widely split first heart sound
    - "v" waves on JVP exam
    - Cool periphery with or without cyanosis
  - EKG: RBBB, tall P-waves, prolonged PR interval
  - ~25% have accessory conduction pathway

- Atrial flutter/atrial fibrillation are common after age 35 years
- Repair indicated especially if:
  - Symptoms of decreased exercise tolerance
  - Worsening tricuspid regurgitation (TR)
  - Cyanosis
- Eisenmenger syndrome:
  - Eisenmenger syndrome develops usually from VSD
  - Leg cyanosis in a patient with PDA → likely from Eisenmenger syndrome physiology
  - Clinical features:
    - Shortness of breath
    - Increased pulmonary arterial pressures
    - Cyanosis
  - Exam:
    - Prominent "a" wave
    - RV heave
    - Palpable and loud P2
    - Ejection click
    - There might be little or even no murmur or might hear a diastolic murmur of PR
- Supravalvular aortic stenosis:
  - Elevated maternal vitamin D levels associated with supravalvular AS
  - Williams syndrome—autosomal dominant
    - More common in males
    - Mental developmental delay
    - Elfin facies
    - Hypercalcemia
  - Exam:
    - Loud systolic murmur over first intercostal space
    - Accentuated A2
    - Right carotid bruit
    - Decreased left brachial pulse
  - Aortic insufficiency can be present; aortic root may be dilated, but there is no associated valvular calcification
  - Indications for surgery:
    - Peak gradient ≥50 mm Hg
    - Mean gradient ≥30 mm Hg

- LV end systolic (ES) diameter ≥50 mm
- Left ventricular ejection fraction (LVEF) <55%
- Patient develops severe and/or symptomatic aortic insufficiency

- Cor triatriatum:
  - Congenital membrane in the left atrium
  - Does not cause mitral regurgitation
  - Can act more like a stenotic lesion—similar to mitral stenosis presentation
- DiGeorge syndrome:
  - Truncus arteriosus
  - Hypocalcemia
- Noonan syndrome:
  - Pulmonic stenosis
  - Webbed neck
  - Ocular abnormalities
- Leopard syndrome:
  - Deafness
  - Pulmonic stenosis
  - Prolonged PR interval
  - Complete heart block
- Kartanager syndrome:
  - Sinusitis
  - Dextrocardia
  - Bronchiectasis
- Holt-Oram syndrome:
  - Autosomal dominant
  - Dysplasia of the upper limbs
  - ASD
- Maternal systemic lupus erythematosus (SLE) can cause congenital heart block
- Fetal alcohol syndrome can be associated with VSD, TOF, and coarctation of the aorta
- Types of cardiac pediatric surgeries to be familiar with:
  - Fontan → there are 3 types:
  - Atriopulmonary connection (the original described procedure)
  - Intracardiac total cavopulmonary connection (lateral tunnel)

- o Extracardiac total cavopulmonary connection
- o Glenn → SVC to PA connection
- o Blalock → subclavian artery to PA connection
- o Waterston → ascending aorta to right PA connection
- o Potts → descending aorta to left PA connection
- Complications after Fontan surgery include:
  - o Sick sinus (bradycardia) is a common arrhythmia
  - o Atrial flutter or atrial fibrillation in the long term
  - o Protein-losing enteropathy

6 Valvular Heart Disease

AORTIC STENOSIS

- Common causes of aortic stenosis include:
  - Calcific AS (mostly in the elderly)
  - Congenital (bicuspid)
  - Rheumatic disease
- Average survival with severe symptomatic aortic stenosis if not treated:
  - Angina—5 years
  - Syncope—3 years
  - Dyspnea/heart failure—2 years
- Bicuspid aortic valve (AV):
  - One of the most common congenital cardiac anomalies
  - More common in men
  - Survival is similar to trileaflet aortic valve
  - Most common bicuspid AV is fusion of right and left cusps
  - Screen first-degree family members
  - Screen entire aorta as these patients have aortopathy
  - Association with aortic coarctation
  - Balloon valvuloplasty outcome of a bicuspid aortic valve is better in kids than in adults:
    - Consider valvuloplasty if symptoms, peak gradient ≥50 mm Hg, and no calcification
    - Consider valvuloplasty if no symptoms and peak gradient is ≥60 mm Hg
  - Surgery for dilated aorta in the setting of bicuspid valve should be considered for aortic diameter of ≥5.5 cm

- In patients <70 years old, ~50% have bicuspid AV with critical aortic stenosis
- Severity of aortic stenosis on exam:
  - Late peaking murmur
  - Absence of S2
  - Paradoxical splitting of S2
  - Pulsus tardus
  - Pulsus brevis
    - NOTE: The loudness of the murmur does not correlate with severity of AS
- Pulse pressure with AS increases after PVC, but pulse pressure decreases with HCM after PVC
- Severe aortic stenosis is defined as:
  - Mean gradient ≥40 mm Hg
  - Jet velocity of 4 m/s
  - Aortic valve area ≤1.0 cm^2
  - Aortic valve area index (calculated as aortic valve area [AVA]/body surface area [BSA]) ≤0.6 cm^2/m^2
- In low-gradient, low LVEF, aortic stenosis, with dobutamine study:
  - True AS → if with ↑ cardiac output, the AV gradient ↑ >40 mm Hg or there is no change in AVA → consider intervention on the valve as this is true aortic stenosis
  - Pseudo AS → if with ↑ cardiac output, the AV gradient is still <30 mm Hg and the AVA increases → for these patients, close observation
- AS with normal LVEF or paradoxical low-flow severe AS:
  - Difficult patient population with restrictive diastolic filling and they can have symptoms of heart failure, angina, or syncope
  - Mean gradient <40 mm Hg
  - Jet velocity <4 m/s
  - Aortic valve area ≤1.0 cm^2
  - Aortic valve area index (calculated as AVA/BSA) ≤0.6 cm^2/m^2
  - Consider surgical aortic valve replacement (SAVR)/transcatheter aortic valve replacement (TAVR) intervention if convinced that symptoms are from aortic valve disease in this condition

- Per American College of Cardiology (ACC)/AHA 2014 guidelines: In asymptomatic patients with AS and a jet velocity ≥4.0 m/s or mean gradient >40 mm Hg, exercise testing can be considered to assess physiological changes with exercise and to confirm the absence of symptoms (stage C)
- In general, timing of surgery (SAVR vs TAVR) for AS:
  - Symptoms
  - If no symptoms, then:
    - LVEF <50%
    - If "fail" exercise stress test (eg, hypotensive response)
- TAVR for symptomatic aortic stenosis has significant survival benefit compared with medical therapy and no surgery
- TAVR and SAVR have similar survival for high-risk and intermediate risk patients
- Risk of stroke with TAVR has reduced with improvement of technology and operator experience to <~2.5%
- Currently, TAVR is indicated for calcific trileaflet aortic valve stenosis. TAVR for bicuspid valve is not Food and Drug Administration (FDA) approved, and current versions of TAVR valves appear to be associated with increased risk of paravalvular leak.
- As opposed to the Edwards valve, the Corevalve cannot be placed via the apical approach
- Approximate risks of TAVR to keep in mind:
  - Pacemaker requirement ~10%
  - Vascular complications 5% to 8%
  - Stroke <2.5%
  - Death <1%

AORTIC REGURGITATION

- Common causes of aortic regurgitation include:
  - Due to valvular disease—for example, bicuspid AV or rheumatic heart disease or endocarditis
  - Due to root/aortic dilation of any cause
- AR should be thought of as whether it is acute vs chronic. If acute:

- Patients are more unstable hemodynamically with pulmonary edema and hypotension due to the sudden increase in LVEDP
- If acute, think of aortic dissection or endocarditis as possible common causes
- Chronic AR is much better tolerated but can lead to LV dilation and dysfunction over time
- Severe aortic regurgitation is defined as:
  - P½ time <200 ms on transthoracic echocardiography (TTE) is severe AR
  - Additional severity indices:
    - Effective regurgitant orifice (ERO) area >0.3 cm^2
    - Regurgitant volume >60 mL
    - Regurgitant fraction >50%
    - Flow reversal in aorta
    - Ratio of (AR color jet dimension) ÷ (left ventricular outflow tract [LVOT] diameter) is >60%
      - NOTE: AR will impact AVA calculation such that the calculated area appears more severe than it actually is
- AR murmur duration (not intensity) correlates with severity. However, in acute severe AR, the diastolic murmur may not even be audible given the rapid rise in the LVEDP and the near equalization with the aortic diastolic pressure
- Wide pulse pressure is noted in chronic AR
- Bisferiens pulse → severe AR
- Timing of surgery for AR:
  - Symptoms
  - If no symptoms, then:
    - LVEF <55%
    - Left ventricular end-systolic diameter (LVESD) >50 mm
    - Left ventricular end-diastolic diameter (LVEDD) >70 mm
- TAVR is not FDA approved for treatment of AR (if stenotic criteria are not met). However, in high-risk nonoperable patients, this has been performed with good results.

MITRAL STENOSIS

- Some causes of mitral stenosis include:
  - Rheumatic
  - Mitral annular calcification
  - Endocarditis
  - Valvulitis (eg, carcinoid—especially if right-to-left shunting is present or pulmonary carcinoid tumor)
  - Congenital
- Increased heart rate/exercise will increase mitral stenosis murmur and make patients more symptomatic
- Cor triatriatum → membrane in the left atrium that might mimic mitral stenosis-type of obstructive physiology
- MS symptoms could include:
  - Shortness of breath/pulmonary edema/pulmonary HTN
  - Atrial fibrillation (likely from dilated LA and increase LA pressure)
  - Stroke/embolic events
- Murmur of MS is a low-pitched diastolic rumble at the apex
- Severity of mitral stenosis:
  - Severe → S2-opening snap is <70 ms
  - Moderate → S2-opening snap is 70 to 110 ms
  - Mild → S2-opening snap is >110 ms
- There is no S3 with mitral stenosis
- MS severity can be defined as:
  - Mean gradient ≥10 mm Hg
  - Pressure ½ time ≥220 ms
  - Mitral valve area ≤1 cm^2
- In addition, MS is severe if:
  - Pulmonary artery systolic pressure (PASP) >50 at rest and >60 mm Hg with exercise
  - Pulmonary capillary wedge pressure (PCWP) ≥25 mm Hg with exercise
- In some patients with mild to moderate MS, symptoms can be managed with heart rate control (goal at rest ~50–60 bpm) and diuretic therapy
- Risk of embolic events with MS is high especially if:
  - Atrial fibrillation is present
  - LA size is >55 mm
  - Spontaneous contrast noted in the LA

- Mitral stenosis valvuloplasty indications:
  - Mitral valve area (MVA) ≤1.5 cm^2
  - Wilkin's score of ≤8
  - PA pressure of >50 mm Hg at rest or >60 mm Hg with exercise
- If valve is not suitable for valvuloplasty, then open surgical intervention should be performed if:
  - Symptomatic MS
  - Consider early intervention if patient is developing atrial fibrillation or pulmonary hypertension from the MS

MITRAL REGURGITATION

- Common causes of mitral regurgitation include:
  - Primary—degeneration of valve leaflet (eg, endo-carditis, MVP, valvulitis, chordal rupture, trauma)
  - Secondary—otherwise known as functional MR (eg, as seen in dilated CMP)
- MVP (Barlow syndrome):
  - Most common cause of MR
  - Prevalence is 1% to 2% of the population
  - Echo definition is prolapse of leaflet of at least 2 mm
  - "Malignant MVP"—with increased risk of malignant arrhythmias:
    - Bileaflet MVP
    - Inverted/biphasic T-waves on EKG
    - Female sex
    - Frequent complex ventricular ectopy
- MR should be thought of as whether it is acute vs chronic. If acute:
  - Patients are more unstable hemodynamically with pulmonary edema and hypotension/shock
  - If acute, think of endocarditis or chordal rupture as possible common causes
  - Chronic MR is better tolerated over time but can lead to LV dilation and dysfunction over time
- MR severity can be defined as:
  - ERO area ≥0.4 cm^2
  - Regurgitant volume ≥60 mL
  - Regurgitant fraction ≥50%

- o Systolic reversal in pulmonary veins
- o Prominent flail MV leaflet or ruptured papillary muscle
- o Vena contracta width ≥0.7 cm with large central MR jet (area <40% of LA) or with a wall-impinging jet of any size, swirling in LA
- MR murmur is a high-pitched holosystolic murmur at apex, which increases with handgrip
  - o If there is posterior papillary dysfunction, the MR jet can be anteriorly directed and MR might best be heard in the precordium
  - o If there is anterior papillary dysfunction, the MR jet can be posteriorly directed and MR might best be heard in the back
  - o In patients with MVP, MR murmur might not be holosystolic and the murmur might begin in mid-systole (after prolapse/mid-systolic click occurs)
  - o In patients with advanced chronic MR, there might be +S3, lateral displacement of the point of maximal impulse (PMI), obscure S1, and possibly widely split S2 (see Table 6.1).

Table 6.1 MR is a volume overload issue and AR is a volume and pressure overload issue

	MR	AR
Preload	↑	↑
Afterload	↓	↑
Ejection fraction (EF) after surgical repair of the valve	↓	=

- If patient with MR has no HTN and preserved LV size and function, there is no benefit of afterload-reducing agents
- Timing of surgery for MR:
  - o Symptoms
  - o If no symptoms, then:
    - LVEF <60%
    - LVESD >40 mm

- Consider early intervention if patient is developing atrial fibrillation or pulmonary hypertension from the MR
- At the present time, MitraClip is FDA indicated for the percutaneous reduction of significant symptomatic mitral regurgitation (MR ≥3+) due to degenerative MR in patients who are too high risk for open mitral valve surgery

ADDITIONAL VALVE ISSUES

- Pulmonary stenosis:
  - 90% of pulmonary stenosis is valvular (not sub- or supravalvular)
  - Associated with Noonan syndrome
  - RV heave, soft late P2, prominent "a" waves in the neck veins, ejection click, and murmur
  - Only right-sided sound that decreases with inspiration → click of pulmonary stenosis
  - The earlier the ejection click, the worse the PS
  - Associated VSD is common with PS (~ two-thirds of cases)
  - Consider valvuloplasty if:
    - Asymptomatic patient if peak and mean gradient are >60 and >40 mm Hg, respectively
    - Symptomatic patient if peak and mean gradient are >50 and >30 mm Hg, respectively
  - If hypotension develops after valvuloplasty, one of the causes to keep in mind is right ventricular outflow tract (RVOT) obstruction due to hypercontraction of the RV when the PS obstruction is removed, and this should be treated not with pressors but rather with volume expansion and beta-blocker therapy
  - Consider open surgery if pulmonic valve is dysplastic
  - If untreated, over time, RV failure can result
- Most common causes of tricuspid regurgitation:
  - Primary—for example carcinoid, Ebstein's anomaly, rheumatic, tumors, endocarditis, radiation
  - Function—for example, dilated RV ± pulmonary HTN, infarct, permanent pacemaker (PPM)

- Prosthetic heart valves:
  - Mechanical valves → ball-cage (Starr-Edwards), disk (Bjork-Shiley; Medtronic-Hall), bileaflet (St Jude's)
  - Bioprosthetic valves → autograft (Ross), homograft, xenograft
- NOTE: The opening click can be heard in a ball-cage valve but not in a bileaflet valve (St Jude valve)
- Anticoagulation goals with warfarin for mechanical prosthetic valves are as follows:
  - Aortic bileaflet valve (St Jude's) or Medtronic-Hall valve → internationalized normalized ratio (INR) goal 2 to 3—in the absence of any other increased/high embolic risk conditions, which include:
    - History of atrial fibrillation/flutter
    - Prior thromboembolic events (on or off anticoagulation)
    - Hypercoagulable states
    - LVEF <30%
  - All other mechanical valves in the aortic position and all mitral mechanical valves or aortic bileaflet/Medtronic-Hall valves in the *presence* of other embolic risk conditions → INR goal is 2.5 to 3.5
- Recommendation for bridging patient's anticoagulation with mechanical valves:
  - This should be considered for essentially all patients except for those with a bileaflet (St Jude's) aortic mechanical valve without any of the increased risk features outlined above
- Aspirin 75 to 100 mg is recommended along with warfarin for all patients with mechanical valve replacement barring any contraindications
- Novel oral anticoagulants are not approved at this time for mechanical valves
- If a patient has none of the high-risk features as listed above and has only a bileaflet aortic valve, you may consider not bridging the patient if he or she needs to come off warfarin for a procedure. All other patients with a mechanical valve should be bridged using either unfractionated heparin (class I) or LMWH (class IIb).

- Hemolysis: ↑ LDH, ↑ bilirubin, ↓↓ haptoglobin, ++ schistocytes
- Least durable valve → Carpentier-Edwards valve
- If a patient has a ball-cage valve (Starr-Edwards), be careful with MRI
- Current indications for endocarditis prophylaxis should be performed in the following subset of patients:
  - Prosthetic heart valves
  - Previous endocarditis
  - Congenital heart disease (eg, unrepaired cyanotic lesion; repair with prosthetic material during first 6 months after device implant; repaired with residual defect)
  - Heart transplant with cardiac valvulopathy
- Antibiotic regimen to consider for endocarditis prophylaxis:
  - Oral amoxicillin (2 g; 30–60 minutes prior to procedure)
  - Intramuscular (IM)/IV ampicillin (2 g) or cefazolin (1 g) or ceftriaxone
  - If allergic to penicillin/ampicillin:
    - Oral cephalexin (2 g), clindamycin (600 mg), or azithromycin or clarithromycin (500 mg)
    - IM/IV cefazolin (1 g), ceftriaxone, or clindamycin
- In general, for gastrointestinal or genitourinary procedures, antibiotic prophylaxis not recommended, but best to check for individual cases/procedures
- For primary prophylaxis for PPM/implantable cardio-verter defibrillator (ICD) placement → use cefazolin (1 g) IV × 1
- In general, staph infections are more common than strep infections for device infections
- Endocarditis of prosthetic valves:
  - Early endocarditis → *Staphylococcus epidermidis*
  - Late endocarditits → *Streptococcus viridans* and/or *Staphylococcus aureus*
- Gram-negative endocarditis most common in patients addicted to narcotics; cirrhosis; prosthetic valves

- Duke's criteria for endocarditis—need 2 major or 1 major and 3 minor or 5 minor criteria to be met for definite diagnosis of endocarditis (Durack, Lukes, Bright 1994; Li, Sexton, Mick, et al. 2000):
  - Major criteria
    - Blood cultures positive (1) typical microorganism for infective endocarditis from 2 blood cultures or (2) persistently positive blood culture defined as 2 positive cultures drawn more than 12 hours apart or 3 to 4 positive blood cultures drawn 1 hour apart or positive single culture for *Coxiella* or antiphase IgG antibody titer >1:800
    - Evidence for endocardial involvement
  - Minor criteria
    - Predisposition
    - Fever
    - Vascular phenomenon
    - Immunologic phenomenon
    - Microbiological criteria that do not meet major criteria
    - Echo minor criteria (this is no longer used in the modified version of the criteria)
- Some peripheral manifestations of endocarditis to be familiar with:
  - Osler's nodes: Tender, red nodules on the hands/feet; likely from immune deposits
  - Janeway lesions: Nontender red lesions on the palms/soles
  - Roth's spots: Retinal bleed with whitish center
- Typical microorganisms for infective endocarditis include viridans streptococci, *Staphylococcus aureus*, *Streptococcus bovis*, HACEK group (see the following point), or community-acquired enterococci in the absence of a primary focus
- HACEK group includes *Haemophilus* species, *Actinobacillus*, *Cardiobacterium hominis*, *Eikenella*, and *Kingella*
- The top 3 gram + cocci to keep in mind include:
  - Viridans strep
  - *Staphylococcus* species
  - *Enterococcus* species

- Transesophageal echocardiography (TEE) (rather than TTE) recommended as first imaging test for workup of endocarditis in the following patients:
  - Prosthetic valve endocarditis
  - Those with at least "possible" endocarditis by clinical criteria
  - Suspected complicated endocarditis, such as paravalvular abscess
- Definition of positive findings on echocardiography for endocarditis:
  - Oscillating intracardiac mass on valve, supporting structures or implanted material
  - Myocardial abscess
  - Dehiscence of prosthetic valve
- TTE is very good at visualizing prosthetic valve aortic regurgitation
- Endocarditis in homeless patients/alcoholic/human immunodeficiency virus (HIV) → *Bartonella* is high on the differential (treat this with erythromycin)
- Patients with poor dental hygiene area at increased risk for HACEK organism endocarditis
- Patient with sheep contact (eg, sheep farmers) are at increased risk for *Coxiella* endocarditis (Q-fever)
- Endocarditis after prostate surgery → enterococcus is high on the differential
- Patients with intravenous drug abuse → increased risk for *S aureus* endocarditis
- *S viridans* endocarditis:
  - 4 weeks for native valve infection
  - 6 weeks for prosthetic valve infection
  - Use penicillin-, ceftriaxone-, and vancomycin-based therapies
- *Staphylococcus* infection endocarditis:
  - 6 weeks for native valve infection → use nafcillin-, cefazolin-, and vancomycin-based therapies
  - For prosthetic valve endocarditis, add rifampin (6 weeks) and gentamycin (2 weeks)
- *Enterococcus* endocarditis:
  - First-line treatment is 4 to 6 weeks of penicillin or ampicillin with gentamycin

- ○ Second-line treatment is ampicillin with ceftriaxone
- HACEK endocarditis:
  - ○ 4 weeks for native valve infections
  - ○ 6 weeks for prosthetic valve infection
  - ○ Use ceftriaxone-, ciprofloxacin-, and ampicillin/ sulbactam-based therapies

7 Heart Failure/Transplant

- Almost half the patients with heart failure (HF) have reduced ejection fraction (HFrEF) and half have preserved ejection fraction (HFpEF)
- Stages of HF include (Hunt, Abraham, Chin, et al. 2005):
  - Stage A—at risk for development of HF but no structural heart disease
  - Stage B—structural heart disease is present but no signs of HF
  - Stage C—structural heart disease with HF symptoms
  - Stage D—refractory HF
- Functional classification of HF (The Criteria Committee of the New York Heart Association 1994):
  - Class I—no symptoms with ordinary activity
  - Class II—symptoms with ordinary activity
  - Class III—symptoms with limited activity
  - Class IV—symptoms at rest
- Some findings to look for on physical exam in patients presenting with HF:
  - Assess if patient is "dry" or "wet"—elevated JVP, peripheral edema, pulmonary edema
  - Assess if patient is "warm" or "cold"—well perfusing or vasoconstricted?
  - Gallop sound (presence of S4/S3)
  - Hepatomegaly/ascites
  - Cheyne-Stokes breathing
  - Abnormal PMI
- Pulsus alternans can be associated with severe left ventricular dysfunction
- Differential diagnosis of HFrEF is long, and some bigger categories of etiologies can include:

- Ischemia
- Infiltrative diseases
- Idiopathic
- Familial
- Tachycardic induced
- Myocarditis/infectious
- Drug toxicity (cocaine/alcohol)
- Chemotherapy side effects
- Stress-induced myopathy
- Autoimmune
- Arrhythmogenic right ventricular dysplasia (ARVD)
- Peripartum
- In HF, there is downregulation of the β1-receptors and not the β2-receptors
- Familial cardiomyopathy (CMP) → up to one-third of idiopathic CMPs
- Hepatomegaly usually precedes edema in congestive heart failure (CHF)
- Annual incidence of HF in diabetic → ~3%/year
- Three-fourths of patients with HF have a history of HTN
- Patients with 3 or more cardiovascular risk factors have ~8%/year risk of HF
- Treatment of HFrEF:
  - Beta-blockers
    - Carvedilol, metoprolol succinate, bisoprolol preferred
    - All patients with reduced LVEF
  - ACE inhibitors
    - Can consider angiotensin receptor blocker (ARB) if ACE inhibitor not tolerated
    - All patients with reduced LVEF
    - No great additive benefit to combine ARB with an ACE inhibitor, and this is not recommended
  - Angiotensin receptor-neprilysin inhibitor (ARNI) (valsartan/sacubitril)
  - Diuretics
    - Loop diuretic
    - Aldosterone antagonist (monitor K level closely)
  - Nitrate-hydralazine
    - Consider in African American patients with New York Heart Association (NYHA) class II to IV symptoms

- - Consider in patients with renal dysfunction and hyperkalemia when an ACE inhibitor/ARB cannot be tolerated
  - Digoxin
    - If this is considered, keep serum digoxin level 0.5 to 1.0 ng/mL
    - Digoxin should not be used in asymptomatic patients with depressed ejection fraction
  - In addition, education in regards to salt and fluid restrictions
  - Avoid these medications:
    - NSAIDs (tramadol may be safer)
    - Calcium channel blockers
    - Thiazolidinediones
- ARNI (valsartan/sacubitril):
  - PARADIGM-HF Trial showed that ARNI reduced cardiovascular mortality and HF hospitalization in HFrEF patients by 20% (McMurray, Packer, Desai, et al. 2014)
    - Class I: Indication in HFrEF
    - Class III: Should not be used concomitantly with ACE inhibitors or within 36 hours of the last dose of an ACE inhibitor/ARB
    - Class III: ARNI should not be administered to patients with a history of angioedema
- Optimize medical treatment prior to considering ICD/ cardiac resynchronization therapy (CRT) placement
- Milrinone increases cAMP levels by inhibition of phospho-diesterase III
- Aliskiren:
  - Decreases renin activity
  - Contraindicated in pregnancy
  - Consider its use in diabetics with HTN
- Indications for CRT:
  - QRS >120 msec and NYHA III
  - QRS >150 msec and NYHA II (ischemic and nonischemic CMP)
  - QRS >150 msec, ischemic CMP, and NYHA I
- Timing of ICD placement on optimal medical therapy:
  - 40 days after MI
  - 90 days after PCI/CABG
  - 90 days after treatment for dilated CMP

- Consider electrophysiology study for ischemic CMP with LVEF 35% to 40% (this does not apply to nonischemic CMP)
- For class IV patients, consider CRT (not just ICD)
- For class I patients, consider ICD for LVEF ≤30%
- HFpEF:
  - ~50% of cases of HF
  - Disease of the elderly
  - Female
  - HTN
  - Obesity
  - Impaired relaxation
  - Diastolic stiffness
  - ↓ e' or the mitral annular velocity during relaxation
  - Atrial fibrillation can be poorly tolerated
  - With diuresis, patients feel much improved rapidly
  - Blood pressure control is important
- Diastolic dysfunction grades:
  - Grade I → delayed relaxation (E/A <1)
  - Grade II → pseudonormal (E/A 1–2)
  - Grade III → restricted (E/A >20)
- Diastolic HF risk increases with age, HTN, obesity, and female sex
- 5-year mortality of HF (similar with preserved and depressed EF) → about 55%
- Diastolic dominant pulmonary vein → diastolic failure; predictor of worse cardiac outcomes (significantly higher rates of HF hospitalizations and cardiovascular death)
- HIV, CD4 <300 is associated with CMP
- High-output HF (eg, thyroid disease, shunts/AV fistulas, anemia, beriberi, Paget disease, pregnancy, carcinoid, multiple myeloma) can result in wide pulse pressure and decreased systemic vascular resistance
- Beriberi:
  - Heart failure
  - Paresthesias
  - Painful glossitis
  - Thiamine deficiency
  - Improvement after thiamine replacement

Essential Facts: Hypertrophic Cardiomyopathy

- Symptoms: Shortness of breath; chest pain; palpitations; syncope/presyncope; fatigue; HF symptoms
- Consider HCM as opposed to athlete's heart if:
  - LVEDD is <45 mm
  - Eccentric hypertrophy
  - No decrease in LV wall thickness with less exercise/deconditioning
  - Left atrial enlargement
  - Abnormal diastolic filling pattern
  - +family history
  - Wall thickness >15 mm
- Histology: Myocardial disarray
- Numerous genes/hundreds of mutations identified mostly on sarcomere gene—some common ones include:
  - B-myosin heavy chain
  - Myosin binding protein
  - Cardiac troponin T
- Autosomal dominant and family screening strongly recommended
- Some notable physical exam findings:
  - S4
  - Bifid pulse
  - Decrease in pulse pressure after PVC
  - Maneuvers that decrease preload, will result in accentuation of the systolic murmur
- Consider treatment if the LVOT peak gradient at rest is >50 mm Hg (especially in symptomatic patients despite medical therapy)
- In HCM, if septum is very thick (>3 cm), septal ablation might not work as well
- Hypotension in HCM should be treated with IV phenylephrine (a pure alpha agonist agent)

(continued)

- Most common arrhythmia: Atrial fibrillation
- Major risk factors for sudden death in HCM (strongly consider ICD placement):
  - Cardiac arrest (ventricular fibrillation [VF])
  - Spontaneous sustained VT
  - Family history of premature
  - Sudden death
  - Unexplained syncope
  - LV thickness ≥30 mm
  - Abnormal exercise BP
  - Nonsustained VT (Holter)
- Avoid strenuous/competitive exercise/sports
- Avoid dehydration
- Alcohol septal ablation results in more RBBB postprocedure
- Surgical myectomy results in more LBBB postprocedure

Essential Facts: Apical HCM

- A variant of HCM with the hypertrophy localized at the cardiac apex
- More common in Asian population
- Giant T-waves in the precordial leads on the EKG may be noted
- Appears to have a more benign prognosis

Essential Facts: Loeffler (Hypereosinophilic) Syndrome

- Apical obliteration
- Thick myocardium from infiltration that results in restrictive filling
- Can also involve the vales and result in MR and/or TR most commonly

Essential Facts: Fabry Disease

- Deficiency of ceramide trihexosidase
- Cardiac infiltration
- ~90% corneal abnormalities/opacities

Essential Facts: Chagas Disease

- RBBB
- Left anterior fascicular block (LAFB)
- Dilated right atrium and bilateral ventricles
- Possible LV apical aneurysm with thrombus

Essential Facts: Anthracycline Risk of CMP

- <1% up to 400 mg/m^2
- ~7% if dosed at 550 mg/m^2

- Doxorubicin can cause endocardial fibrosis
- Busulfan can cause pulmonary fibrosis and endocardial fibrosis
- Ifosfamide can result in HF
- LV noncompaction:
  - Prominent LV trabeculae
  - Increased risk of cardioembolic events
  - HF can occur
  - Echo and especially MRI very helpful for diagnosis
  - Treatment of HF symptoms and barring contraindications, consider anticoagulation
  - Consider recommending against competitive sports
- Pompe disease (type II glycogen storage disease):
  - CMP with tall QRS and short PR interval
  - Failure to thrive
- If patient has dilated CMP and HTN → rule out pheochromocytoma

Essential Facts: Amyloid Cardiomyopathy

- Restrictive CMP
- Age of presentation ~60 years
- More commonly male
- AL primary amyloid (multiorgan; 50% cardiac)
- Low volts on EKG
- Biventricular hypertrophy on echo
- Avoid digoxin
- Diurese for HF
- Poor prognosis of <1 year with AL amyloid, ~2 to 3 years with mutation in transthyretin (TTR), and ~5 years with senile form of amyloid
- Isolated LA cardiac amyloid with no other organ involvement may be considered for cardiac transplant combined with stem cell transplant

Essential Facts: Sarcoid Cardiomyopathy

- Noncaseating granuloma
- Clinical cardiac sarcoid is ~5% but autopsy cardiac involvement in sarcoid patients is 40% to 50%
- AV block and ventricular arrhythmias
- Abnormal cardiac MRI with patchy delayed gad enhancement
- PET scan abnormal with increased FDG uptake in areas of inflammation
- Cardiac biopsy can be considered but it is low yield given patchy nature of cardiac involvement
- Treatment with diuresis; treating underlying sarcoid; PPM for AV block might be needed

- Mortality on LVAD is <~10% at 30 days; a low mean pulmonary pressure is a predictor of poor outcome after LVAD
- Some indications for cardiac transplant include:
  - Hemodynamic compromise due to HF
  - Refractory cardiogenic shock

- Dependence on IV inotropic support
- Peak VO_2 of <10 mL/kg/min
- Severe symptoms of ischemia limiting routine activity
- Recurrent symptomatic ventricular arrhythmias refractory to all therapy

---

Essential Facts: Cardiac Hemochromatosis

- Primary (hereditary) vs secondary (blood transfusion)
- Hereditary form is autosomal recessive
- More common in Eastern European
- More common in middle-aged male patients
- Conduction disorder
- Other organs may be involved:
  - Joints
  - Liver
  - Testes
  - Endocrine organs
  - Skin with "bronze diabetes"
- Liver biopsy can be considered for diagnosis
- Laboratory findings: ↑ ferritin and iron/total iron binding capacity (TIBC) ratio >50%
- Cardiac MRI abnormal with reduced T2 signal
- Treatment with phlebotomy/chelation

- Some contraindication to cardiac transplant include:
  - Malignancy
  - Active infection
  - Irreversible pulmonary hypertension despite therapy
  - Active substance abuse
  - Lack of social support or lack of medical compliance
  - Relative contraindications might include older age, other end-organ failure
- After 1 year of cardiac transplantation, the number 1 cause of death is cancer and the number 2 cause of death is vasculopathy
- Humoral rejection after heart transplant (otherwise known as vascular rejection) is antibody-mediated

(B-cell) → pending severity of rejection, consider treatment
with plasmapheresis, steroids, intravenous gamma-
globulin, antithymocyte antibodies, and/or rituximab
- Posttransplant lymphoproliferative disease → B-cell
lymphoma
- T-cell rejection is most common after heart transplant → treat with steroids and increase immune
suppression
- Risk of cytomegalovirus (CMV) after heart transplant is
highest with CMV+ donor and CMV—recipient → treat
with IV ganciclovir followed by prolonged therapy
- Epstein-Barr virus (EBV)–negative patients are at
increased risk for posttransplant lymphoproliferative
disease (B-cell lymphoma)
- Consider treating transplant vasculopathy with:
  ○ Higher antiproliferative immunosuppressants
  ○ ↓ steroids dosing
  ○ Aggressive statin use
- Calcineurin inhibitors include cyclosporine, tacrolimus → with these agents, careful with renal toxicity and
hemolytic uremic syndrome

Essential Facts: Cyclosporine
- Levels are increased with ketoconazole and
erythromycin and the levels are decreased with
phenytoin and phenobarbital
- Side effects → gingival hyperplasia, hirsutism,
tremor
- Verapamil, cardizem, and nicardipine can ↑ cyclosporine levels

- Tacrolimus side effects → glucose intolerance, tremor
- Azathioprine side effects → hepatic dysfunction; also be
careful as it interacts with allopurinol
- Rapamycin side effects → increases lipids; oral lesions;
wound-healing issues
- Mycophenolate mofetil side effects → gastrointestinal
intolerance; increased risk of viral infection

8 Acute Coronary Syndromes

- Troponin I (not troponin T) is more specific to diagnose acute coronary syndrome (ACS) in renal failure
- ~10% to 15% of patients with ACS have no significant angiographic CAD
- In women, plaque erosion is more common in those <50 years old and plaque rupture more common in those >50 years old
- In men, plaque rupture more common at all ages than plaque erosion
- For every 30-minute delay in reperfusion for ST-elevation myocardial infarction (STEMI), the risk of mortality at 1 year increases by ~7%
- For every 1% increase in HDL, there is a 2% decrease in coronary events
- Original Sgarbossa criteria for diagnosing STEMI in the presence of LBBB (Smith, Dodd, Henry, et al. 2012):
  - Concordant ST elevation ≥1 mm in a lead with a positive QRS complex (5 points)
  - Discordant ST elevation ≥5 mm in a lead with a negative QRS complex (2 points)
  - ST depression ≥1 mm in lead V1, V2, or V3 (3 points)
    - (≥3 points = >90% specificity of STEMI but sensitivity is <50%)
- TIMI risk score for unstable angina/NSTEMI includes (Antman, Cohen, Bernick, et al. 2000):
  - Age ≥ 65 years
  - ≥3 CAD risk factors
  - Known CAD (stenosis ≥50%)
  - Aspirin use in past 7 days
  - Severe angina (≥2 episodes in 24 hours)

- ○ EKG ST changes ≥0.5 mm (note: NOT T-wave inversion)
  - ○ Positive cardiac biomarker
- Thrombolysis in myocardial infarction (TIMI) risk score 6 to 7 → 14-day death/MI/revascularization ~40%
- TIMI risk score 0 to 1 → 14-day death/MI/revascularization ~4.7% (Table 8.1)

Table 8.1 TIMI risk score for STEMI

	Points
Age	
65–74	2
≥75	3
Diabetes/HTN or angina	1
SBP < 100	3
HR > 100	2
Killip classes II to IV	2
Weight < 67 kg (147.7 lbs)	1
Anterior ST ↑ or LBBB	1
Time to treatment > 4 hours	1

Source: Morrow, Antman, Charlesworth, et al. 2000.

- Estimated odds ratio of death at 30 days:
  - ○ 0.1 for score 0
  - ○ 1.2 for score 4
  - ○ 8.8 for score >8
- TIMI risk score for STEMI of (Morrow, Antman, Charlesworth, et. al. 2000):
  - ○ 0 to 2 → mortality 1% to 2%
  - ○ 3 to 4 → mortality 4% to 6%
  - ○ 5 to 6 → mortality 10% to 15%
  - ○ ≥7 → mortality ≥20%
- GRACE score includes the following (Fox, Dabbous, Goldberg, et al. 2006):
  - ○ Age
  - ○ Killip class (Table 8.2)
  - ○ Systolic blood pressure
  - ○ Heart rate

- ○ Serum creatinine
- ○ ST segment elevation
- ○ Cardiac arrest on admission
- ○ Positive cardiac biomarkers

Table 8.2 Killip classification

Mortality		
Class I	No CHF	6%
Class II	+S3 and basilar crackles on exam	17%
Class III	Pulmonary edema	30%–40%
Class IV	Cardiogenic shock	60%–80%

Source: Killip and Kimball 1967.

- Consider early invasive strategy for NSTEMI for:
  - ○ Recurrent angina or ischemia at rest or with low-level activities despite intensive medical therapy
  - ○ Elevated cardiac biomarkers (TnT or TnI)
  - ○ New or presumably new ST-depression
  - ○ Signs or symptoms of heart failure
  - ○ Hemodynamic instability
  - ○ High risk score (eg, GRACE, TIMI)
  - ○ Sustained ventricular tachycardia
  - ○ PCI within 6 months
  - ○ Prior CABG
  - ○ Diabetes mellitus
  - ○ Mild to moderate renal dysfunction
  - ○ Reduced LV function (LVEF <40%)
- Absolute contraindications to lytic therapy:
  - ○ Any prior intracranial hemorrhage
  - ○ Known structural cerebral vascular lesion (eg, arteriovenous malformation)
  - ○ Known malignant intracranial neoplasm (primary or metastatic)
  - ○ Ischemic stroke within 3 months except acute ischemic stroke within 3 hours
  - ○ Suspected aortic dissection
  - ○ Active bleeding (excluding menses)

- Significant closed-head trauma or facial trauma within 3 months
- Relative contraindications to lytic therapy:
  - History of chronic, severe, poorly controlled hypertension
  - Severe uncontrolled hypertension on presentation (SBP >180 mm Hg or DBP >110 mm Hg)
  - History of ischemic stroke greater than 3 months, dementia, or known intracranial pathology not covered in contraindications
  - Traumatic or prolonged (>10 minutes) CPR or major surgery (<3 weeks)
  - Recent (<2 to 4 weeks) internal bleeding
  - Noncompressible vascular punctures
  - For streptokinase/anistreplase: prior exposure (>5 days ago) or prior allergic reaction to these agents
  - Pregnancy
  - Active peptic ulcer
  - Current use of anticoagulants: the higher the INR, the higher the risk of bleeding
- Doses of lytic agents for STEMI:
  - Streptokinase: 1.5 million units over 30 to 60 minutes
  - tPA: 15-mg bolus and then 0.75 mg/kg (maximum 50 mg) over 30 minutes
  - rPA: 10 U bolus ×2 (30-minute agent)
  - Tenecteplase (TNK):
    - Weight <60 kg → 30 mg
    - Weight 60 to 69 kg → 35 mg
    - Weight 70 to 79 kg → 40 mg
    - Weight 80 to 89 kg → 45 mg
    - Weight ≥90 kg → 50 mg
- Streptokinase
  - Least fibrin specific
  - Depletes fibrinogen levels the most
  - Half-life is 20 minutes
- TNK is the most fibrin specific of the lytic agent
- tPA has a short half-life of 5 to 10 minutes in the body
- TNK = tPA in regards to mortality; TNK associated with less bleeding compared with tPA (ASSENT-2 Trial)

- To reverse the action of lytics, consider treating with:
  - Cryoprecipitate
  - Fresh-frozen plasma
  - And/or epsilon aminocaproic acid
- STEMI patients presenting to a non-PCI hospital should be transferred to a PCI capable center even after successful lysis
- Shock Trial → significant mortality benefit at 6 months (but NOT at 30 days) (SHOCK Investigators, Hochman, Sleeper, et al. 1999; Hochman, Sleeper, Webb, et al. 1999)
- In cardiac arrest patients, for every hour of delay in initiating cooling, there is ~20% increased risk of death
- Treat cardiogenic shock with vasopressin
- 5-FU can increase risk of MI
- Best predictor of mortality in shock is cardiac power, calculated as:
  - (MAP × cardiac output [CO])/451
- Argatroban is hepatically metabolized
- Tirofiban is renally metabolized
- Bivalirudin (Angiomax):
  - ~25-minute half-life
  - <25% removed with dialysis
  - Do not use this for conservative therapy of NSTEMI
- Avoid fondaparinux in renal failure (if glomerular filtration rate [GFR] <30)
- Abciximab (Reopro) has a ~2% risk of thrombocytopenia and this risk doubles if patients are reexposed to this medication within 2 weeks
- Complications post-MI to keep in mind:
  - Ventricular septal defect (VSD)
    - VSD is more common with first myocardial infarction, older patients, female, hypertensive, and much more common with an anterior MI (more apical VSD) vs inferior MI (more basal VSD)
    - Post-MI VSD has poor prognosis but it is worse with basal septal VSD
  - Free wall rupture
    - Free wall rupture most commonly associated with left circumflex territory MI, older age, use of steroids, HTN
  - Papillary muscle rupture

- Papillary muscle rupture/acute MR most commonly associated with older age, female, and inferior MI
  - LV thrombus
  - Ventricular aneurysm
  - Arrhythmias (AF, VT, accelerated idioventricular rhythm; heart block)
    - Mobitz II more common with an anterior MI
    - Consider placing temporary pacing wire during MI if alternating BBB is present with high-grade block
  - Pericarditis
  - Dressler syndrome
- Mortality post-MI—some numbers to keep in mind:
  - 30-day mortality post-MI is about ~1%
  - 1-year mortality post-MI is about ~3%
  - 5-year mortality post-MI is about ~7% to 8%
- Inability to exercise post-MI has a bad prognosis
- Cardiac rehab has been associated with ~25% reduction of cardiac mortality post-MI
- Academic Research Consortium (ARC) definition for stent thrombosis (Table 8.3):

Table 8.3 Timing of ARC definition for stent thrombosis

Acute	<24 hours
Subacute	24 hours to 30 days
Late	>30 hours
Very late	>12 months

Source: Cutlip, Windecker, Mehran, et al. 2007.

  - Definite: Angiographic confirmation of a thrombus in the stent (or within 5 mm of each edge of the stent) or pathologic confirmation of stent thrombosis
  - Probable: Unexplained death within 30 days after the procedure or MI in an area supplied by the stented vessel but without angiographic confirmation of stent thrombosis
  - Possible: Unexplained death more than 30 days after the procedure

- Very late stent thrombosis → think of stent malapposition
- Late or subacute stent thrombosis (rather than very late thrombosis) → think of stent length and bifurcation stenting issues
- Stent underexpansion:
  - ↑ risk of Instent restenosis (ISR)
  - ↑ risk of thrombosis
- ACS presentation does not predict ISR
- Approximate incidence of coronary stent thrombosis on dual antiplatelet therapy is 0.5% to 1.5%
- Long-term management after ACS:
  - Aspirin 81 mg daily (lifelong)
  - DAPT (clopidogrel, prasugrel, or ticagrelor) (at least 1 year)
  - Beta-blocker
  - Lipid-lowering therapy with high-intensity statin
  - ACE inhibitor (ACEI) or ARB especially for patients with CHF, LV dysfunction (EF <0.40), hypertension, or diabetes
  - Aldosterone blockers (eplerenone) for patients with LVEF <40% and CHF
  - Smoke cessation and lifestyle modifications as indicated
- Prasugrel:
  - Contraindicated in patients with history of stroke/ TIA
  - Not recommend for patients ≥75 years old
  - Care with patients who are <60 kg—can consider a lower maintenance dose of 5 mg daily (rather than 10 mg daily)
- Ticagrelor:
  - Rapid onset
  - Not a prodrug (unlike clopidogrel and prasugrel)
  - Side effects might include dyspnea, ventricular pauses
  - Aspirin dose should be <100 mg when used in combination with ticagrelor
- Cangrelor:
  - Intravenous P2Y12 inhibitor
  - Active drug

- ○ Indicated for PCI
- ○ Not indicated at this time as "bridge" therapy prior to surgical procedures
- ○ Transition to oral P2Y12 inhibitors as follows:
  - Ticagrelor at any time during infusion of cangrelor or immediately after discontinuation
  - Prasugrel and clopidogrel—immediately after discontinuation of cangrelor (these should not be given during cangrelor infusion as drugs interact)
- Additional management issues to consider after ACS:
  - ○ Influenza vaccination
  - ○ Screening for depression and treating as indicated
  - ○ Avoidance of NSAIDs
  - ○ Avoidance of hormone replacement therapy
  - ○ Avoidance of antioxidant vitamin supplements (eg, vitamins E and C or beta-carotene)
  - ○ Avoidance of folic acid, with or without B6 and B12
- Risk factors for postmyocardial VSD development:
  - ○ Older age
  - ○ Female
  - ○ History of hypertension
  - ○ No history of smoking
  - ○ Killip classes III to IV
- On MRI, myocardial scar results in late gadolinium enhancement and appears bright
- Timing of ICD placement after ACS on optimal medical therapy is ≥40 days after MI

9 Pericardial Disease

- Normal pericardial thickness ~2 mm
- Congenital absence of the pericardium can be associated with:
  - Bradycardia
  - ASD
  - Bicuspid AV
  - Bronchogenic cyst
- Some causes of pericarditis/effusion:
  - Infectious (eg, viral, bacterial, tuberculosis [TB], fungal) <5% of the time
  - Neoplastic <10% of the time
  - Uremia
  - Radiation induced
  - Autoimmune/rheumatologic conditions (eg, connective tissue disease such as lupus/rheumatoid arthritis, vasculitis)
  - Drug induced
    - Procainamide
    - Hydralazine
    - Methylsergide
    - Minoxidil
    - Isoniazid (for tuberculosis treatment)
  - Idiopathic ~90% of the time
- EKG changes in pericarditis:
  - Diffuse ST elevation
  - Diffuse PR depression
  - PR elevation in aVR
- Lytic therapy for acute MI can decrease risk of post-MI pericarditis

- Most common fungal pericarditis is due to histoplasmosis
- TB pericarditis results in 30% to 50% constriction physiology and is associated with high mortality
- Pain associated with pericarditis is positional (better sitting forward)
- Most common pericardial tumor in adults is mesothelioma
- Most common pericardial tumor in infants is teratoma
- Pericardial cysts:
  - Uncommon (<0.1%) congenital anomaly
  - Often asymptomatic and incidentally found on imaging study
  - Management options might include observation, cyst drainage, and/or surgical removal pending symptoms and location of cyst
- Physical exam of pericarditis might be associated with a pericardial rub, but if an effusion is present, this might not be heard and the heart sounds might be very distant
- Pericardial rub has 3 phases:
  - Atrial systole
  - Ventricular systole
  - Ventricular diastole
- EKG with a large pericardial effusions may show low volts and electrical alternans (beat-to-beat variation of QRS amplitude)
- Beck's triad on physical exam for tamponade includes:
  - Distant heart sounds
  - Elevated JVP
  - Hypotension
- Pulsus paradoxus is a SBP drop of ≥10 mm Hg with inspiration
- One of the findings on the physical exam in tamponade is dullness to percussion of the left lung base (this is known as Evant's sign)
- SVR is typically elevated in tamponade as the body's compensation to perfuse organs; cardiac output is decreased

- Pericardial tamponade without pulsus can be seen when aortic regurgitation is present or with a large ASD or with severe rheumatoid spondylitis
- There is interdependence of the ventricles with cardiac tamponade
- Tamponade physiology on echocardiography exists when the difference between the highest and the lowest velocity across the mitral or tricuspid valve is more than 25%. Also note diastolic RA and RV collapse and dilated IVC without respiratory variations.
- Echocardiographic diagnosis of tamponade in patients with pulmonary HTN can be challenging given increased right-sided intracardiac pressures and RVH
- For pericardiocentesis, be careful not to drain more than 1 L acutely as there is some risk for acute RV dilation. Of note, a pattern of LV stress myopathy has also been observed with large-volume pericardiocentesis.
- Pericardial effusion after heart surgery can occur over 50% of the time with risk of tamponade ~1% to 2%; this can occur ~1 week postoperatively
- Pericardial effusion is rare in rheumatoid arthritis but the glucose level can be low and the rheumatoid factor elevated in this fluid
- Tamponade, in the absence of a pericardial effusion, can be caused from outside compression of the cardiac chambers (eg, a mass/tumor)
- Tamponade physiology can be present in the absence of a large pericardial effusion if the fluid is loculated and/or compressing one of the cardiac chambers only (eg, after cardiac surgery/loculated effusion)
- Treatment of pericarditis is with high-dose NSAIDs (eg, ibuprofen 600–800 mg 3x/daily or aspirin 800–1000 mg 3x/daily) for a 1- to 2-week course in addition to colchicine (0.5 mg twice daily) x 3 months. Note that proton pump inhibitors (PPIs) are best used along with the above to decrease the risk of gastrointestinal (GI) side effects.
- Steroids not first-line therapy for pericarditis—can consider for systemic autoimmune/rheumatologic conditions

- Diagnostic yield from pericardial effusion fluid is low. The yield is much better if one obtains pericardial tissue at the time of surgical pericardial window placement.
- Equalization of mean right atrial pressure, right ventricular ejection fraction (RVEDP), pulmonary capillary wedge pressure, and blunted y-descent in the RA tracing is highly suggestive of tamponade
- If after pericardiocentesis the pericardial pressure has decreased but the RA pressure remains elevated, consider effusive-restrictive pericardial process
- Constrictive pericarditis can occur in 1% to 2% of the cases of pericarditis of any cause
  - Have increased level of suspicion in patients with prior radiation therapy to the chest, Hodgkin disease, prior cardiac surgery, or breast cancer
- Some drugs that can cause constrictive pericarditis:
  - Procainamide
  - Hydralazine
  - Methylsergide
- Kussmaul sign → increase or lack of decrease in the JVP with inspiration. This is noted in constrictive pericarditis but can also be seen in RV failure/infarct, tricuspid stenosis, or cor pulmonale.
- Some physical exam findings that might be present in constrictive pericarditis:
  - Kussmaul sign
  - Prominent y-descent
  - Hepatomegaly
  - Ascites
  - Edema
  - Pericardial knock
- Brain natriuretic peptide (BNP) in constrictive pericarditis is typically not elevated, whereas this is elevated in restrictive cardiomyopathy
- If septal bounce is noted on echocardiography, consider constrictive pericarditis
- Mitral annular velocity with tissue Doppler is elevated with constriction (>20 cm/s is severe)

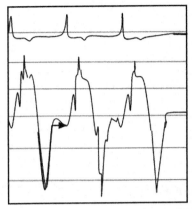

Figure 9.1 Dip and plateau configuration in RV filling in constriction and restriction.

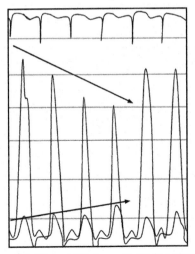

Figure 9.2 LV and RV discordance in constrictive pericarditis.

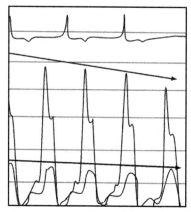

Figure 9.3 LV and RV concordance in restrictive
cardiomyopathy.

- Invasive atrial tracing in constrictive pericarditis and
  restrictive CMP might show prominent x- and
  y-descents (otherwise known as the "M" or "W" sign)
- Dip and plateau configuration in the RV filling can be
  seen in constriction and restriction (Figure 9.1)
- Right ventricular systolic pressure is usually >55 mm Hg
  in restrictive CMP and <55 mm Hg in constrictive
  pericarditis
- Ventricular (LV and RV) discordance is present in
  constrictive pericarditis (Figure 9.2), whereas concordance is present in restrictive CMP (Figure 9.3). This
  has a sensitivity of ~100% and specificity of ~95%.
- Treatment of constrictive pericarditis is to gently
  diurese, and if the pericardium is very thickened on CT
  or MRI (>~4mm), consider surgical pericardiectomy
- Treatment of restrictive CMP will depend on the etiology
  of the restriction/infiltrative process

10 Electrophysiology

- Phases of cardiac action potential (Table 10.1)

Table 10.1 Phases of cardiac action potential

Phase 0	Upstroke/rapid depolarization Rapid Na^+ influx
Phase 1	Early rapid repolarization K^+ efflux by opening of the transient K^+ channel
Phase 2	Plateau Influx of Ca^{++} balanced with efflux of K^+
Phase 3	Final rapid repolarization Ca^{++} close but delayed rectifier K^+ remain open
Phase 4	Diastolic depolarization Na^+ and Ca^{++} channels close; open K^+ rectifier channels keep the transmembrane potential to −90 mV

- Normal AH interval → 60 to 120 ms
- Normal HV interval → 35 to 60 ms
- Ventriculo-atria (VA) interval of <70 ms is short
- Resting potential for AV nodal cells is −40 to −70 mV
- Electrophysiological study is poor at evaluating sinus node dysfunction
- Differential diagnosis for bradycardia/heart block:
  - Sinus bradycardia
  - First-degree AV block (with PR > 200 ms)
  - Second-degree AV block:
    - Mobitz 1 (Wenckebach)—due to AV node conduction delay

- ■ Mobitz 2—due to His-Purkinje conduction delay
  - ○ Third-degree block
- Acquired AV block—some causes:
  - ○ Idiopathic
  - ○ CAD/infarction
  - ○ Calcific valvular disease
  - ○ Infectious
    - ■ Lyme
    - ■ Syphilis
    - ■ Chagas
  - ○ Infiltrative
    - ■ Sarcoid
    - ■ Amyloid
    - ■ Hemochromatosis
  - ○ Neuromuscular
  - ○ Collagen vascular disease
    - ■ Scleroderma
    - ■ SLE
    - ■ Dermatomyositis
    - ■ Rheumatoid arthritis
  - ○ Drug effect
    - ■ Digoxin
    - ■ Beta-blocker
    - ■ Calcium channel blocker
    - ■ And other AV nodal blocking agents
- In an asymptomatic patient with congenital third-degree heart block, consider PPM placement if:
  - ○ Pauses of >3 seconds
  - ○ Decline in exercise tolerance
  - ○ Widening of the QRS interval
  - ○ CMP
  - ○ Increase in QT length
- Chronotropic incompetence is a class I indication for PPM placement
- Differential diagnosis for SVT:
  - ○ Regular:
    - ■ Sinus tachycardia
    - ■ Atrial tachycardia
    - ■ Atrioventricular nodal reentrant tachycardia (AVNRT)

- - Atrioventricular reentrant tachycardia (AVRT)
  - Atrial flutter with regular block (often 2:1 at rate of 150 bpm)
  - ○ Irregular:
    - Atrial fibrillation
    - Atrial flutter with variable block
    - Multifocal atrial tachycardia
- Adenosine or vagal maneuvers terminate reentrant AVRT and AVNRT
- Atrial tachycardia terminates in "V"
- AVNRT/AVRT terminates in "A"
- Incidental WPW → obtain echocardiogram to rule out Ebstein's anomaly and other structural heart disease
- Wide complex irregular tachycardia → consider AF with WPW. Use procainamide or ibutillide and avoid calcium channel blockers or pure AV nodal blocking agents.
- Location of accessory pathways in WPW can be figured according to Table 10.2.

Table 10.2 Wolff-Parkinson-White accessory pathways

	V1	aVF	aVL
Left lateral	+	+	−
Left posterior/septal	+	−	+
Right posterior/septal	−	−	+
Right lateral/anterior	−	+	+

Source: Friberg, Rosenqvist, Lip 2012.

- Some etiologies for atrial fibrillation:
  - ○ Cardiac (heart failure, cardiac surgery, myocarditis, valvular heart disease, etc)
  - ○ Pulmonary (COPD)
  - ○ Metabolic (stress/elevated catecholamine/pheochromocytoma/thyroid disease)
  - ○ Drugs (alcohol/amphetamines/cocaine)
  - ○ Neurogenic (stroke/cranial bleed)
- CHADS-VASC2 score for stroke risk factors (January, Wann, Alpert, et al. 2014) (see Table 10.3)

Table 10.3 CHADS-VASC2 score

	Score
Congestive heart failure (or left ventricular systolic dysfunction)	1 point
HTN (treated hypertension on medication)	1 point
Age ≥75 years	2 point
Diabetes mellitus	1 point
Prior stroke or TIA or thromboembolism	2 points
Vascular disease (eg, peripheral artery disease, myocardial infarction, aortic plaque)	1 point
Age 65 to 74 years	1 point
Female sex	1 point

Annual risk of stroke per CHADS-VASC2 score

Score 0	0%	Score 5	~6.7%
Score 1	~1%	Score 6	~9%
Score 2	~2%	Score 7	~10%
Score 3	~3%	Score 8	~12%
Score 4	~4%	Score 9	~15%

Source: Lip 2011.

- Anticoagulation recommended for CHADS-VASC2 score of ≥2; might consider antiplatelet therapy and/or anticoagulation for score of 1 pending risk of bleeding (can use HAS-BLED risk calculator below).
- HAS-BLED score for the risk factors for bleeding (see Table 10.4)
- Anticoagulation options for AF:
  - Warfarin (INR goal 2–3)
  - NOACs – at this time NOAcs are not indicated for AF due to severe mitral stenosis
    - Factor Xa inhibitors (rivaroxaban, apixaban, edoxaban)
    - Direct-thrombin inhibitor (dabigatran).
- Consider electrical cardioversion or pharmacologic therapy for first-time AF patients. If AF is >48 hours,

Table 10.4 HAS-BLED score

	Score
Scoring	
Hypertension (>160/90 mm Hg)	1 point
Abnormal renal/liver function	1 point each
Stroke	1 point
Bleeding/predisposition to bleeding	1 point
Labile INRs	1 point
Age >65 years	1 point
Drugs/NSAIDs	1 point
Alcohol	1 point
Risk of bleeding per score	
Low risk (1.1%)	0–1 points
Moderate risk (~2%)	2 points
High risk (~4.9%)	≥3 points

perform TEE to rule out left atrial appendage (LAA) clot prior to cardioversion. Otherwise, anticoagulate for 3 to 4 weeks and then cardiovert. After cardioversion, anticoagulation should be continued for minimum of 4 weeks.
- Sotalol not helpful for cardioversion
- Propafenone (600 mg orally ×1) helpful with cardioversion
- Consider LAA closure by surgical closure vs Lariet device vs Watchman device if patient not great candidate for anticoagulation but high risk for stroke
- Pulmonary vein ablation for AF best considered for patients with paroxysmal AF. Success rate ~80%. Some complications of this procedure include:
  - Bleeding
  - Pulmonary vein stenosis
  - Stroke
  - Pericarditis/tamponade
  - Phrenic nerve injury
  - LA-esophageal fistula
- For treatment of atrial fibrillation, consider:

- ○ Vagally associated AF → consider treatment with disopyramide
- ○ If patient is in heart failure → consider using amiodarone
- ○ If patient has CAD → consider using sotalol/dofetilide/ amiodarone
- ○ If patient has LVH ≥ 1.4 cm → consider using amiodarone
- ○ If patient has structurally normal heart → consider using propafenone/fleicanide/sotalol/amiodarone
- ○ If patient is on dialysis, do not use sotalol or dofetilide
- There is less risk of atrial fibrillation with atrial or AV sequential pacing compared to VVI or VVIR pacing (refer to Table 10.5 on page XX below)
- Consider PPM in patients with atrial fibrillation if pauses >5 seconds when awake
- Catheter ablation in AF improves quality of life and symptom relief but does not decrease hospitalization
- In nonvalvular AF, the LAA is the source of clot in ~90% of cases
- Early after depolarization—example of arrhythmia:
  - ○ Torsade de pointes
- Delayed after depolarization—example of arrhythmia:
  - ○ Digoxin-induced arrhythmias
  - ○ RVOT VT
- Some causes of ventricular tachycardia:
  - ○ Monomorphic VT:
    - Prior MI/scar
    - CMP
    - RVOT VT
    - LV VT
    - Fascicular/papillary muscle VT
    - ARVD
    - Idiopathic VT
    - Ischemia (more commonly polymorphic VT)
    - HCM
    - Myocarditis (consider giant cell)
  - ○ Polymorphic VT:
    - Ischemic CMP
    - Brugada syndrome
    - Long QT

- Congenital channelopathies
- Torsades de pointes
- Catecholaminergic polymorphic ventricular tachycardia (CPVT)

- VT criteria on EKG:
  - AV dissociation—100% VT
  - Capture beat—100% VT
  - Fusion beat—100% VT
  - Extreme axis—right superior axis with + R-wave in aVR
  - Additional Brugada criteria for VT:
    - Concordance in the precordial leads (leads V1–V6)
    - R to S interval >100 ms in any one precordial lead
    - Morphology of the QRS complex as follows:
      – If RBBB pattern is present, VT diagnosis if:
        □ A monophasic R or biphasic qR complex in V1
        □ If an RSR' pattern is present in V1 with the R peak being higher in amplitude than the R' peak, then VT is present
        □ rS complex in lead V6 favors VT
      – If LBBB pattern is present, VT diagnosis if:
        □ Presence of any Q- or QS-wave in lead V6 favors VT
        □ A wide R-wave in lead V1 or V2 of 40 ms or more favors VT
        □ Slurred or notched downstroke of the S-wave in V1 or V2 favors VT
        □ Duration of onset of the QRS complex to peak of QS- or S-wave >60 ms favors VT
- Wide complex tachycardia in a patient with a scar from prior MI is very likely (>90% of the time) to be VT
- Brugada syndrome:
  - Sodium channel loss of function
  - Placing EKG lead V1/2 higher up on the chest might bring out Brugada pattern of RBBB
  - Avoid bupivacaine
- QT prolongations could be due to numerous causes (eg, some psychiatric medications, antimicrobials, antiarrhythmics, or due to hypocalcemia, hypothermia, hypothyroidism, bradycardia, bundle branch block, cardiomyopathy)

Essential Facts: ARVD

- More common in males than females
- ARVD is autosomal dominant
- Due to mutation in desmosome
- EKG → epsilon waves; QRS might be a bit wider in V1 than V6
- Infiltration of RV by fat
- Echo and MRI can be very helpful for making diagnosis
- Combination of 2 major, a major, and 2 minor criteria or 4 minor criteria
- Some major criteria:
  - Severe dilation and reduction of RVEF with mild or no LV involvement
    - Localized RV aneurysm (akinetic or dyskinetic areas with diastolic bulging)
  - Severe segmental RV dilation
- Some minor criteria:
  - Mild global RV dilation and/or reduction with normal LV
  - Regional RV hypokinesis
  - Late potentials on signal-averaged EKG
    - Inverted T-waves in right precordial leads (in V1 through V3 above age 12 years, in the absence of RBBB)
  - LBBB VT (sustained or nonsustained) on EKG, Holter, or ETT
  - Frequent PVCs (>1000/24 hours on Holter)
  - Family history of premature sudden death (age <35 years) due to suspected ARVC
  - Family history of clinical diagnosis based on present criteria
- Treatment of heart failure and consideration of ICD ± VT ablation

- Long QTS:
  - Loss of function of voltage-gated potassium channel (IKs/IKr) in two-thirds of patients
  - ICD for aborted cardiac arrest
  - Family history not as predictive in long QT syndrome (LQTS)
  - Most drug-induced long QT is the binding to the IKr receptor

---

Essential Facts: Long QT Subtypes

- Long QT1
  - 30% to 35% of cases
  - Exercise-triggered events (eg, swimming)
  - Wide-based QT
  - Consider treating with ICD and beta-blocker (either nadolol or propranolol; not atenolol or metoprolol)
- Long QT2
  - 25% to 35% of cases
  - Auditory stimuli-triggered events
  - Double-hump QT
  - More common in females
  - Postpartum
- Long QT3
  - 5% to 10% of cases
  - Event during sleep
  - Prolonged ST-segment
  - Sodium channel leakiness
  - Consider treating with ICD
  - Controversial whether sodium channel blocker (eg, mexiletine) may be helpful

---

- Jervell-Lange-Nielsen syndrome → long QT, autosomal recessive, deafness
- Romano-Ward syndrome → long QT, autosomal dominant, no deafness
- Torsades de pointes (due to prolong QT) therapies:

- ○ IV magnesium therapy
- ○ Increasing the heart rate will shorten the QT interval, so consider temporary pacing, IV isoproterenol, or both
- ○ Unsynchronized cardioversion beginning with 100 Joules
- ○ Lidocaine shortens the QT interval and may be effective especially for drug-induced torsades de pointes
- ○ Avoid class Ia, Ic, and III antiarrhythmics
- RVOT VT:
  - ○ LBBB morphology to the VT with inferior axis
  - ○ Often after exercise
  - ○ Can sometimes use calcium channel blocker as therapy
  - ○ Invasive of ablation of VT is also an option
- Bidirectional VT usually caused by:
  - ○ Digoxin toxicity
  - ○ CPVT
- CPVT:
  - ○ Due to leaky ryanodine receptor
  - ○ Alterations in calcium channel release in sarcoplasmic reticulum
  - ○ Autosomal dominant
  - ○ Exercise triggered
  - ○ Premature ventricular contraction (PVC) may initiate CPVT at HR > 120 bpm
  - ○ ICD recommended for cardiac arrest
  - ○ Controversial whether verapamil or flecainide might be useful
  - ○ Of note, flecainide appears to decrease ryanodine receptor
- Fascicular VT:
  - ○ More common in males
  - ○ Typically younger age
  - ○ RBBB
  - ○ Can occur with exercise or rest
  - ○ Treatment:
    - Verapamil (not beta-blocker)
    - Ablation

- Bundle branch reentry VT should be considered in patients with dilated CMP
- 5-year mortality in patients with syncope:
  - Cardiac cause → ~19% to 30%
  - Noncardiac cause → ~6%
- Syncope with exertion of the upper extremity → think about subclavian steal syndrome
- Syncope with movement of neck/head and/or tying a necktie/scarf with neck motion → think about carotid sinus hypersensitivity
- Syncope with rapid onset and with premonition → think about vasovagal syncope
- Placement of a pacemaker in hypertrophic obstructive cardiomyopathy (HOCM) appears to decrease LV systolic dimension but does not change LV diastolic dimension
- Pacemaker infections:
  - Early: *Staphylococcus aureus*
  - Late: *Staphylococcus epidermidis*
- Optimize medical treatment prior to considering ICD/ CRT placement
- Indications for CRT:
  - QRS > 120 ms and NYHA III
  - QRS > 150 ms and NYHA II (ischemic and nonischemic CM)
  - QRS > 150 ms, ischemic CMP, and NYHA I
- Timing of ICD placement on optimal medical therapy:
  - 40 days after MI
  - 90 days after PCI/CABG
  - 90 days after treatment for dilated CMP
- Consider electrophysiology study for ischemic CMP with LVEF 35% to 40% (this does not apply to nonischemic CMP)
- For class IV patients, consider CRT (not just ICD)
- For class I patients, consider ICD for LVEF ≤ 30%
- Atrioventricular synchrony with PPM decreases risk of atrial fibrillation
- If a patient has tachy-brady atrial fibrillation → use VVI (R) mode of PPM

- Neurocardiogenic syncope → consider DDD pacing (which is superior to VVI pacing in this condition)
- Pacemaker codes (see Table 10.5)
- Pacemaker-induced tachycardia → treat by increasing the PVARP (postventricular atrial refractory period)
- Drugs that block sodium channels → ↑↑ pacing threshold
- For PPM interrogation, keep the following in mind (see Table 10.6)

Table 10.5 Pacemaker codes

First letter	Chamber paced
Second letter	Chamber sensed
Third letter	Response to sensed beat
Fourth letter	Program feature
Fifth letter	Antitachycardia functions

Note: A, atrial; V, ventricular; O, none; I, inhibited; T, triggered; D, dual; R, rate modulation.

Table 10.6 PPM Interrogation

Wire fracture	High-voltage threshold; high impedance
Lead dislodgement	High-voltage threshold; normal impedance
Insulation break	Low-voltage threshold; low impedance
Exit block	High-voltage threshold; normal impedance
Lead perforation	Increased lead impedance

11 Pharmacology

- β_1 stimulation → ↑ heart rate (HR) and ↑ contractility
- α_1 stimulation → ↑ preload and ↑ afterload
- β_2 stimulation → ↓ afterload

Table 11.1. Agonists and antagonists for β_1, α_1, and β_2 receptors

Examples of agonists	
Phenylephrine (Neo)	α agonist
Isoproterenol	β_1 and β_2 agonist
Norepineprhine (Levo)	90% α agonist; 10% β_1 agonist (NOTE: lacks β_2, but stronger α-stimulant)
Epinephrine	50% α agonist and 50% β_1 and β_2 agonist
Examples of antagonists	
Phentolamine/prazosin	α_1 antagonist
Propranolol/metoprolol	β_1 and β_2 antagonist
Labetalol	α_1, β_1, and β_2 antagonist

- Elimination route for common cardiovascular drugs:
  - Hepatic: amiodarone; propafenone; lidocaine; mexilitine; verapamil; diltiazem
  - Renal: sotalol; digoxin; dofetilide; bretylium; atenolol; N-acetylprocainamide (NAPA)
  - Mixed hepatic and renal: procainamide; flecainide; quinidine; ibutilide
- Dronaderone should not be used for CHF or chronic AF
- Avoid using dofetilide:

○ With verapamil, cimetidine, ketoconazole, trimethoprim
○ If QTc > 440 ms (or 500 ms with an ICD)

Table 11.2. Classification of antiarrhythmic drugs

Class I	Block fast sodium channels
○ IA	○ ↓ Vmax → quinidine/disopyramide/ procainamide → ↑QT
○ IB	○ Vmax → mexilitine/lidocaine/phenytoin → ↓↓ (shorten) action potential (↓ QT)
○ IC	○ ↑Vmax → propafenone/fleicanide → ↑QRS/ PR → "use dependent"
Class II	Beta-blockers
Class III	Amiodarone/sotalol/dofetilide → block potassium channels (IKr and not IKs) → ↑QT → "reverse use dependent" (which means most affect at slower heart rates)
Class IV	Block calcium channels

Essential Facts: ACE Inhibitor/ARB

- If creatinine level increases over 35% from baseline, consider holding this
- Decreased effectiveness if used along with NSAIDs
- No effect on lipids
- Avoid during pregnancy (side effects might include low birth weight, early delivery, oligohy-dramnios, neonatal anemia, and renal failure)
- Can be considered postpartum but not during pregnancy
- ACE inhibitors can cause taste disturbance and cough
- Should not be used concomitantly with ARNI

- Grapefruit juice inhibits CYP3A—careful with drug interactions (eg, statins, calcium channel blockers, cyclosporine, amiodarone, cilostazol)

Essential Facts: Statins

- Antibiotic daptomycin can increase the risk of rhabdomyolysis if patient is taking a statin
- Statins can rarely cause pancreatitis
- Grapefruit juice can interact with statins (eg, simvastatin, lovastatin)
- SLCO1B1 (which is a hepatic drug uptake transporter) polymorphism may be a risk factor for statin-induced side effects, especially in simvastatin therapy
- St John's Wort can decrease the bioavailability of statin
- Statins metabolized by CYP3A4 → simvastatin/lovastatin/atorvastatin
- Statins metabolized by CYP2C9 → fluvastatin/rosuvastatin
- Pravastatin is not metabolized by CYP450
- In Asian patients, start rosuvastatin at low dose of 5 mg daily
- In renal failure, use either atorvastatin or fluvastatin
- Simvastatin should be used carefully in combination with these medications due to muscle toxicity:
  - Maximum dose of 10 mg when used in combination with amiodarone/diltiazem/verapamil
  - Maximum dose of 20 mg when used in combination with amlodipine/Ranexa

- St John's Wort can decrease the bioavailability of certain medications (eg, calcium channel blockers, statins, β-blockers, and amiodarone)
- HIV medications:
  - Protease inhibitors in HIV treatment affect the lipid level
  - Nucleosome reverse transcriptase inhibitors (eg, abacavir or didanosine) increase risk of MI

Essential Facts: Beta-Blockers

- Can cause bronchospasm
- Can increase triglyceride levels
- Hydrophilic beta-blockers are renally excreted (eg, atenolol and sotalol) and do not cross blood-brain barrier
- Lipophilic beta-blockers are hepatically cleared (eg, metoprolol, labetolol, and propranolol) and cross blood-brain barrier
- Pindolol → non-cardioselective beta-blocker with intrinsic sympathomimetic activity (ISA)
- Acebutolol → selective beta-blocker with intrinsic sympathomimetic activity
- Bisoprolol → β_1-selective
- For beta-blocker toxicity, IV glucagon can increase both the SA and AV nodal conduction
- For beta-blocker overdose, consider treating with glucagon and milrinone

Essential Facts: Diuretics

- Thiazide diuretic can increase LDL and triglyceride levels
- Loop diuretics can cause hypocalcemia and decrease renin level
- Thiazide diuretics/metolazone (Zaroxolyn) can cause hypercalcemia
- Thiazide diuretics do not decrease renin level
- Acetazolamide (Diamax) → can cause metabolic acidosis

- Haloperidol can cause increased QT interval and torsade de pointes
- Clozapine can cause postural hypotension
- Phenytoin can cause gingival hyperplasia
- Disopyramide can cause urinary retention

Essential Facts: Digoxin

- Digoxin's ionotropic effects are via inhibition of the sodium-potassium ATPase and sodium-calcium exchange
- Delayed after depolarization (as opposed to ibutilide, for example)
- Not dialyzable; if need be, consider using Digibind for digoxin toxicity
- Hawthorn berry can increase digoxin effect
- Many drugs can interact with digoxin and increase its levels (eg, quinidine, propafenone, amiodarone, verapamil, cyclosporine, antifungal agents, etc)
- Digoxin should not be used in asymptomatic patients with depressed ejection fraction
- Digoxin toxicity can cause numerous arrhythmias—including bidirectional VT, heart block, regularization of atrial fibrillation
- Avoid cardioversion in digoxin toxicity
- $\downarrow K^+ / \downarrow Ca^{++} \rightarrow$ increase risk of digoxin toxicity

Essential Facts: Amiodarone

- Prodrug and is not dialyzable
- Can cause pulmonary toxicity, thyroid side effects, and hepatitis, but in addition, ~10% of the time peripheral neuropathy
- Diarrhea is not associated with this medication
- Amiodarone can interact with warfarin, digoxin, and cyclosporine → and result in ↑ levels of all of these drugs
- Amiodarone can ↑ DFT (defibrillation threshold) (as opposed to sotalol which ↓ DFT) despite the fact that both are class III antiarrhythmic agents
- Can be used during pregnancy

- Dopamine is contraindicated in patients with MAO inhibitors
- G6PD deficiency is a contraindication for quinidine use
- Keep the following in mind when using IV adenosine:
  - Careful if patient is also taking dipyridamole (as it has an increased effect)
  - Careful if patient is following heart transplant (as it has increased effect)
  - If patient is on theophylline, the adenosine dose might have to be increased or you might want to avoid this agent

Essential Facts: Quinidine

- Side effects may include nausea, vomiting, anorexia, and diarrhea
- Thrombocytopenia/bone marrow suppression
- Fever
- Rare reports of SLE
- Dose-independent arrhythmias can occur
- Stop quinidine if QRS width ↑ by 25% or QT >550 ms
- Careful with interaction with other meds:
  - Digoxin/phenytoin/rifampicin/phenobarbitol all ↓ quinidine level
  - Ketoconazole ↑ quinidine level
  - Quinidine can ↑ digoxin level

Essential Facts: Propafenone

- Metabolized via CYP450 2D6 enzyme
- Keep in mind that ~70% of the US population lacks this enzyme
- ↑ Digoxin/warfarin and Lopressor levels
- ↑ QRS and ↑ PR interval

Essential Facts: Procainamide

- Can result in ~20% to 30% SLE; ~25% GI side effects
- 60% to 70% of patients develop antibodies to procainamide
- Can also result in fever, granulocytosis
- Dose-independent arrhythmias can occur
- Careful with its use if patients have underlying bundle branch block or intraventricular conduction delays

Essential Facts: Ibutilide

- 2% to 3% risk of torsade de pointes
- Upon initiation of this medication, keep patient in the hospital for ~24 hours for observation
- If the LVEF is <20%, risk of this medication is higher
- Early after-depolarization (as opposed to digoxin, for example)

Essential Facts: Lidocaine

- Can cause seizure
- Decrease dose with liver disease; clearance is not renal
- Decrease clearance of lidocaine with prolonged infusion
- Toxicity can occur with 8 to 10 hours of treatment

- Flumazenil → dose 0.2 mg (maximum 1 mg); onset 6 to 10 minutes
- Naloxone → dose 0.4 mg (maximum 2 mg); onset 5 to 10 minutes
- Bupivacaine is anesthetic with high risk for cardio-vascular toxicity

- Chantix (varenicline):
  - Start this medication ~1 week prior to target quit date of smoking
  - Nausea is a main side effect
  - If neuropsychological side effects, stop the drug

12 Pregnancy

- Pregnancy is associated with the following changes:
  - Increased intravascular volume
  - Increased cardiac output
  - Increased heart rate
  - Decreased systemic vascular resistance (SVR)
- Physical exam findings that are due to normal changes of pregnancy:
  - Soft systolic murmur
  - +S3
  - Widely split and loud S1
- Physical exam findings that are abnormal during pregnancy:
  - S4
  - Loud (≥ 3/6) systolic murmur or diastolic murmurs
  - Fixed split S2
- Conditions that pregnancy should be advised against include:
  - Severe pulmonary HTN
  - Severe mitral stenosis with MVA < 2 cm^2
  - Severe aortic stenosis with AVA < 1.5 cm^2
  - Aortic disease:
    - Coarctation of the aorta
    - Dilated aorta (eg, Marfan with an aorta > 4–4.5 cm)
  - HCM
  - Ventricular dysfunction, especially class III/IV symptoms, or LVEF < 40%
  - History of peripartum CMP, especially if the LVEF has not recovered
  - Severe cyanosis

- MI in pregnancy—consider the following in your differential:
  - Coronary artery dissection (more common in third trimester)
  - Cocaine/drug abuse
  - Risk is much higher if hypercoagulable state is present (such as antiphospholipid antibody syndrome [APLS])
- Rubella infection in mother during pregnancy can be associated with:
  - Pulmonary artery stenosis
  - PDA
  - Pulmonary stenosis
  - VSD
  - ASD
  - Tetralogy of Fallot
  - Coarctation of the aorta
    - But no association with Ebstein's
- Dipyridamole (Persantine) is contraindicated in pregnancy
- Warfarin in first trimester of pregnancy might result in nasal hypoplasia, microcephaly, mental developmental delay, optic neuropathy
  - Risk highest during weeks 6 to 12 of pregnancy
  - The risk is lower if < 5 mg daily dose is used
- Anticoagulation in pregnancy:
  - Recommendation continues to be controversial and larger randomized prospective studies are needed to address this issue
  - First trimester: warfarin, low molecular weight heparin (LMWH), intravenous unfractionated heparin (UFH) (all dose adjusted)
  - If using LMWH, consider weekly monitoring with peak and trough anti-factor Xa levels to assure therapeutic efficacy and patient compliance—keep trough ≥ 0.6 IU/ml for low risk patients and ≥ 0.7 IU/ml for high risk patients and peak < 15 IU/ml.
  - 2 to 3 weeks prior to delivery → change to intravenous UFH

- Higher heparin doses might be required during pregnancy due to increased plasma volume and more heparin-binding protein
- Some medical conditions to consider C-section during pregnancy:
  - Severe pulmonary HTN
  - Patient on warfarin
  - Dilated or enlarging aorta (≥~4 cm)
  - Severe stenotic valvular lesions where sudden change in blood pressure might be of concern
- Peripartum cardiomyopathy:
  - Risk factors: age > 30 years, twin pregnancy, African American, multiparous
  - ~50% improve at 6 months; ~20% normalize LVEF
  - Mortality ~10% at 6 months and ~25% at 2 years
  - Recurrence is ~20% with normal rest LVEF but abnormal LVEF with exercise
  - Recurrence is double (~40%) with abnormal rest LVEF
  - Repeat pregnancy should be discouraged if LVEF remains abnormal after initial event
  - ↑ levels prolactin; ↑ cathepsin D; ↑ angioplastic 16-kDa prolactin
  - In addition to typical heart failure treatments, consider therapy with bromocriptine to suppress prolactin level → 2.5 mg BID × 2 weeks then daily
  - Also, consider using anticoagulation if LVEF is < 35% given increased risk of LV thrombus formation in the hypercoagulable postoperative period
- Sotalol, flecainide, lidocaine, procainamide, amiodarone can be used during pregnancy
- Consider treating HTN in pregnancy with:
  - Methyldopa (first-choice agent)
  - Long-acting nifedipine (second-choice agent)
- Fetal alcohol syndrome and rubella infection in the mother during pregnancy is associated with TOF

13 Pulmonary Hypertension

- Pulmonary hypertension (HTN) is defined as:
  - Mean pulmonary arterial pressure ≥25 mm Hg at rest usually confirmed by right heart catheterization
- Presenting symptoms might include:
  - Shortness of breath
  - Right-sided heart failure
  - Decreased exercise tolerance
- World Health Organization (WHO) classifications (Table 13.1 and Table 13.2)
- Prevalence of pulmonary HTN is 1 in 200 HIV-infected patients. This is ~ 10 times greater than non-HIV patients. This prevalence does not appear to have changed since antiretroviral therapy.

Table 13.1 WHO classification of pulmonary hypertension

Group 1	PAH (idiopathic, familial, connective tissue disease, HIV, portal HTN, congenital heart disease, schistosomiasis)
Group 2	PH due to left heart disease (ventricular or valvular abnormalities)
Group 3	PH due to chronic lung disease and/or hypoxemia (interstitial lung disease, pulmonary fibrosis, emphysema, obstructive sleep apnea)
Group 4	Chronic thromboembolic pulmonary hypertension (CTEPH)
Group 5	Chronic thromboembolic pulmonary hypertension (CTEPH)

Source: Simonneau, Robbins, Beghetti, et al. 2009.

Table 13.2 WHO functional classification of symptoms

Class I	Asymptomatic with ordinary activities
Class II	Symptoms with ordinary activity
Class III	Symptoms with minimal activity
Class IV	Symptoms at rest

Source: Simonneau, Robbins, Beghetti, et al. 2009.

- Presence of pericardial effusion is a bad prognostic sign in pulmonary hypertension (PH)
- Some likely physical exam findings in pulmonary HTN:
  - Loud P2
  - Right-sided gallop sound
  - RV heave
  - Pulmonary flow murmur
  - Elevated JVP
  - Edema/ascites/hepatomegaly
- ↓ diffusing capacity of the lungs for carbon monoxide (DLCO) with pulmonary HTN
- TAPSE (tricuspid annular plane systolic excursion) > 18 mm (normal). If RV dysfunction is present with pulmonary HTN, TAPSE might be decreased.
- PA pressure alone correlates poorly with outcome
- 6-minute walk test is useful in assessment of patients with PH; generally, if patients can walk:
  - < 300 m severe condition
  - 300 to 500 m moderate condition
  - > 500 m mild condition
- Echocardiographic findings of RV pressure and volume:
  - Pressure overload: Flattened septum in systole
  - Volume overload: Flattened septum in mid-to-late diastole
- RVOT Doppler pattern (see Figure 13.1, p. 102)
- Bone morphogenetic protein receptor 2 (BMPR2) gene and its product transforming growth factor β (TGF-β) receptor appear to have a role in pulmonary arterial hypertension (PAH)

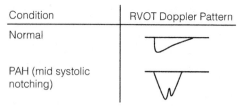

Figure 13.1 RVOT Doppler pattern in normal vs PAH.

- Vasodilator response in PH is positive if there is a:
  - ↓ mean pulmonary artery pressure (mPAP) ≥ 10 mm Hg
  - ↓ mPAP to ~40 mm Hg
  - Only ~10% with PH are vasodilator positive
- Busulfan can cause pulmonary fibrosis and endocardial fibrosis
- Chronic thromboembolic pulmonary hypertension (CTEPH):
  - V/Q scan best noninvasive modality for diagnosis
  - Pulmonary angiogram best invasive test for diagnosis
  - Consider surgery for more definitive therapy
- Patients with pulmonary HTN with PVR >7 Woods units and those with pulmonary vascular resistance (PVR)/ SVR ratio of > two-thirds are very high risk
- Therapy for pulmonary HTN:
  - Supportive care (oxygen, diuretic)
  - Consider digoxin if RV dysfunction
  - Anticoagulation
  - Treat underlying causes of pulmonary HTN
  - Vasodilator therapy (choice of agent based on severity of condition)
    - If patient is vasoreactive, you can consider using a calcium channel blocker
    - If patient is not vasoreactive and functional class III/IV, consider using IV epoprastenol (which is an IV prostacycline)
    - If patient is not vasoreactive and functional class I/II, many agents are available (eg, sildenafil, bosentan, ambrisentan, tadalafil, etc)

- In patients with pulmonary arterial HTN who present with angina, obtain a coronary computed tomography angiogram (CTA) to evaluate for left main (LM) compression from an enlarged pulmonary artery (PA) (Galie N, Sais F et al.2017)
  - Almost 40% of patients with pulm HTN with anginal symptoms have been reported to have LM compression
  - Best predictor of LM compression is a PA diameter of ≥ 40 mm.
  - Therapeutic options for such LM compression is either surgical or percutaneous coronary stenting
- For acute RV failure:
  - Consider IV dobutamine
  - Inhaled nitric oxide (NO)
- Vasoactive agent classes:
  - Calcium channel blockers (nifedipine; careful with diltiazem if RV failure is present)
  - Prostacycline analogues:
    - IV epoprastenol
    - Iloprost (inhaled)/treprostinil (IV or subcutaneous [SC])/selexipag
  - Endothelin receptor antagonists:
    - Nonselective agents (both receptors A and B): bosentan, macitentan
    - Selective for receptor A: ambrisentan, sitaxsentan
  - PDE-5 inhibitor (sildenafil, tadafil)
  - Guanylate cyclase stimulator (to increase cGMP) (riociguat)
- Keep some toxicities in mind:
  - Epoprastenol → flushing, jaw/leg pain, nausea
  - Bosentan → liver toxicity; teratogenic; ↓ efficacy of estrogen contraceptive
  - Ambrisentan → less abnormalities in the liver function tests
- Some risk factors for poor prognosis:
  - 6-minute walk test of <300 meters
  - RV failure
  - Class IV symptoms

- o Increased RA pressure (>20 mm Hg) and low cardiac index (<2.0 L/min/kg)
  - o Elevated BNP
  - o Pericardial effusion
- Keep in mind that right-to-left shunting might occur with elevated right-sided pressures in the setting of a PFO
- For severe pulmonary HTN and right heart failure, despite aggressive advanced therapy and maximal diuretic therapy, lung transplantation and/or atrial septostomy might be considered, but the latter is likely to worsen right-to-left shunting
- 3-year survival is ~48% after diagnosis

14 Peripheral Vascular Disease

ANEURYSM

- Aortic aneurysm is defined as >3 cm; aortic ectasia is defined as > 2.5 cm
- Abdominal aortic aneurysm (AAA):
  - More common in males than females
  - Most significant risk factor is family history of AAA
    - 10% to 15% of AAAs are familial
  - Screening as follows:
    - Asymptomatic men ≥60 years who are siblings or offspring of AAA patients (class I; level of evidence [LOE] B)
    - Asymptomatic men aged 65 to 75 years who have ever smoked (class IIa; LOE B)
    - Patients presenting with a palpable/pulsatile abdominal mass
- Thoracic aortic aneurysm is as common in both sexes, but the risk of rupture is higher in females
- Treatment of patients with aneurysm includes:
  - BP treatment
  - Smoking cessation
  - Statin therapy
  - Screening with noninvasive imaging (computed tomography [CT], MRI, or abdominal US [if AAA])
    - If size is <4 cm, then imaging every 2 to 3 years
    - If size is 4 to 5 cm, then at least yearly imaging
  - For AAA—consider surgical intervention for diameter of ≥5.5 cm or if the size is increasing by ≥0.5 cm/y
    - Rupture rate for AAA >5.5 cm is >~10%/y

- ○ For thoracic aortic aneurysm (TAA)—consider surgical intervention for diameter of ≥ 5.5 cm or even ~5 cm if there is a positive family history and/or connective tissue disease/Marfan and/or if the size is increasing by ≥0.5 cm/y
- Endovascular repair (EVAR) of abdominal and thoracic aneurysm depends on aortic anatomy and the overall risk of surgery to the patient based on comorbidities. EVAR for AAA is associated with decreased length of stay, less bleeding, and possibly lower short-term mortality, but long-term endograft leak and need for reintervention are higher—close imaging follow-up and surveillance are required.
- Types of aortic dissection:
  - ○ If ascending aorta involved:
    - Stanford A
    - DeBakey I (involves ascending and descending aorta)
    - DeBakey II (involves ascending aorta only)
  - ○ If only descending aorta involved:
    - Stanford B
    - DeBakey III
- Some risk factors for aortic dissection:
  - ○ Older age
  - ○ HTN
  - ○ Male sex
  - ○ Smoker
  - ○ Connective tissue disease/Marfan/Ehlers-Danlos
  - ○ Aortitis (eg, syphilis, Takayasu)
  - ○ Coarctation of the aorta/Turner
  - ○ Bicuspid aortic valve with enlarged aorta
  - ○ Trauma
  - ○ Drug use (eg, cocaine)
- Ascending aortic dissection should be managed emergently surgically. Risk of death is ~1%/h in the first 48 hours. Watch out for acute aortic regurgitation, pericardial effusion, and extension of the dissection into the coronary arteries.
- Descending aortic dissection can be managed medically or, if complications arise, then surgically

(either open surgery or endovascular approach). Some complications of descending aortic dissection to monitor include poor perfusion to the legs/gut/spine. Serial follow-up imaging for unoperated dissection should be considered with CT/MRI at 1, 3, and 6 months and then annually.
- Loeys-Dietz syndrome: aortic aneurysm, bifid uvula, cleft palate, hypertelorism (wide-set eyes)
- Intracranial aneurysms are associated with family history/hereditary, smoking, HTN, aortic coarctation. Most commonly found incidentally.
  - If symptomatic, they need to be repaired
  - If asymptomatic and ≥ 7 mm, consider repair
  - If <7 mm, can be observed with CT/MRI imaging every 6 months. If stable, can screen every 2 years.

PERIPHERAL ARTERY DISEASE

- In patients with PAD, annual risk of MI/stroke/vascular death is ~5%
- 5-year cardiovascular mortality in patients with PAD is ~20%
- Diabetic patient with chronic limb ischemia:
  - ~40% chance of gangrene
  - ~15% chance of amputation
- Classification systems (Tables 14.1, 14.2, 14.3, and 14.4)
- Peripheral arterial disease screening:

Table 14.1 Rutherford classification

Stage 0	Asymptomatic
Stage 1	Mild claudication
Stage 2	Moderate claudication
Stage 3	Severe claudication
Stage 4	Rest pain
Stage 5	Minor tissue loss with ischemic nonhealing ulcer or focal gangrene with diffuse pedal ischemia
Stage 6	Major tissue loss—extending above transmetatarsal level, functional foot no longer salvageable

Source: Rutherford, Baker, Ernst, et al. 1997.

Table 14.2 Fontaine classification

Stage I	Asymptomatic
Stage II	Intermittent claudication
○ Stage IIa	○ Intermittent claudication after more than 200 meters of pain-free walking
○ Stage IIb	○ Intermittent claudication after less than 200 meters of walking
Stage III	Rest pain
Stage IV	Ischemic ulcers/gangrene

Source: Fontaine, Kim, Kieny 1954.

Table 14.3 TASC II Classification of femoral and popliteal lesions

Type A lesions	○ Single stenosis ≤ 10 cm in length
	○ Single occlusion ≤ 5 cm in length
Type B lesions	○ Multiple lesions (stenoses or occlusions), each ≤ 5 cm
	○ Single stenosis or occlusion ≤ 15 cm not involving the infrageniculate popliteal artery
	○ Single or multiple lesions in the absence of continuous tibial vessels to improve inflow for a distal bypass
	○ Heavily calcified occlusion ≤ 5 cm in length
	○ Single popliteal stenosis
Type C lesions	○ Multiple stenoses or occlusions totaling > 15 cm with or without heavy calcification
	○ Recurrent stenoses or occlusions that need treatment after two endovascular interventions
Type D lesions	○ Chronic total occlusion of the common or superficial femoral artery (> 20 cm, involving the popliteal artery)
	○ Chronic total occlusion of the popliteal artery and proximal trifurcation vessels

Source: Norgren, Hiatt, Dormandy, et al. 2007.

Table 14.4 ABI classification

Normal	0.9–1.3
Mild	0.7–0.9
Moderate	0.5–0.7
Severe	0.3–0.5

- ○ Exertional leg symptoms or rest pains (typically including the forefoot), usually associated with diminished or absent pulses, which become increasingly severe with elevation and diminish with placement of the leg in a dependent position
- ○ Nonhealing wounds
- ○ Patients with circulatory disorders who are at high risk with abnormal pulse exam
- ○ Adults > 65 years of age
- ○ Adults > 50 years of age with diabetes or tobacco use
- • Ankle-brachial index (ABI) > 1.3 to 1.4 is likely due to arterial calcification/noncompressibility and not diagnostic. This can occur in patients with diabetes or renal dysfunction on hemodialysis.
- • Normal TBI (toe-brachial index) is > 0.7
- • Treatment of PAD includes:
  - ○ Smoking cessation
  - ○ Exercise program
  - ○ Statins
  - ○ Antiplatelet therapy
  - ○ ACE inhibitor/angiotensin receptor blocker therapy
  - ○ HTN control
  - ○ Diabetes control
  - ○ Revascularization—method of revascularization will depend on anatomy and local expertise:
    - ▪ Surgical
    - ▪ Endovascular
    - ▪ For below-the-knee PAD in a claudicant without any critical limb ischemia (CLI), medical therapy preferred option at this time

- Patency rates are highest for both surgical and endovascular therapies in the iliac system (5-year patency ~80%)

Essential Facts: Cilostazole
- PDE3 inhibitor
- ↑ cAMP
- Inhibits platelet β-selection

- Revascularization (open surgical or endovascular) for chronic PAD depends on the anatomy and clinical presentation
- The 6 "Ps" of acute limb ischemia:
  - Pain
  - Pallor
  - Paresthesias
  - Pulselessness
  - Paralysis
  - Poikilothermia or polar (cold leg)
- Acute limb ischemia is a surgical emergency. Etiologies to consider:
  - Embolic (eg, atrial fibrillation or other cardioembolic or aortic sources)
  - Trauma
  - Heparin-induced thrombocytopenia/thrombosis and/or hypercoagulable states (antiphospholipid antibody syndrome) and/or stent thrombosis
- Acute limb ischemia:
  - 30-day mortality ~15%
  - Amputation rate ~15% to 30%
- Baker cyst typically is associated with pain behind knee, knee stiffness, and pain with prolonged standing and worse with bending. In absence of vascular disease, ABI is normal.
- Vasculitis classification:
  - Large vessel
    - Giant cell arteritis
    - Takayasu arteritis

- o Medium vessel
  - Polyarteritis nodosa
  - Kawasaki disease
- o Small vessel
  - Antineutrophil cytoplasmic antibody (ANCA)–associated vasculitis
    - Churg-Strauss
    - Granulomatosis with polyangiitis (Wegener)
    - Microscopic polyangiitis
  - IgA vasculitis (Henoch-Schönlein purpura)
  - Cryoglobulinemic vasculitis
  - Cutaneous leukocytoclastic angiitis
- Kawasaki disease can cause rash in childhood in the palms/soles
- Churg-Strauss—keep in mind associations with:
  - o Asthma
  - o Allergies
  - o Nasal polyps

Essential Facts: Giant Cell Arteritis

- Headache
- Myalgias
- More common in females
- Elevated ESR
- Spares branch vessels

Essential Facts: Takayasu Arteritis

- Age >40 years
- Does not spare branch vessels—there can be a blood pressure difference between the arms of 10 (or more) mm Hg
- Possible bruit over the subclavian artery
- Claudication of an extremity
- Angiography can show narrowing of aorta and branches

Essential Facts: Polyarteritis Nodosa
- ANCA-negative medium-vessel vasculitis
- Patient may have systemic symptoms and multiorgan involvement such as skin lesions with palpable purpura, weight loss, renal dysfunction, joint pain, and neurologic and GI tract involvement
- More common in males
- Middle-aged or older patients (usually peak is in sixth decade of life)
- Most cases are idiopathic but some might be associated with hepatitis B/C and hairy cell leukemia
- Biopsy for confirmation of diagnosis

Essential Facts: Granulomatosis With Polyangiitis (Previously Known as Wegener Granulomatosis)
- ANCA-associated small-vessel vasculitis
- Granulomatous inflammation of the respiratory tract
- Necrotizing pauci-immune glomerulonephritis

Essential Facts: IgA Vasculitis (Henoch-Schönlein Purpura)
- Usually in children
- Abdominal and joint pain
- Rash (small, red to purple, slightly raised areas)
- Renal involvement

Essential Facts: Thromboangiitis Obliterans (Buerger Disease)

- Strongly associated with smoking
- Recurring/progressive inflammation and clotting of small- and medium-sized vessels
- Pain
- More common in younger males
- Amputation risk is > 2 times higher in the patients who continue to smoke

STROKE

- Carotid artery disease screening:
  - Patients with a history of stroke or TIA
  - Patients who are scheduled for coronary artery bypass graft (CABG) surgery and meet one or more of the following criteria: age greater than 65 years, presence of left main coronary artery stenosis, peripheral artery disease, history of smoking, history of TIA or stroke, or presence of a carotid bruit
  - Carotid artery disease is more prevalent in patients with PAD compared with CAD
- Other risk factors for carotid artery disease:
  - FMD
  - Vasculitis
  - Radiation therapy
  - Dissection (in patients with HTN)
- Normal peak systolic velocity of vertebral arteries is 20 to 60 cm/s
  - If > 100 cm/s → severe stenosis
- Carotid duplex is inferior to magnetic resonance angiogram (MRA) if:
  - High carotid bifurcation
  - Long (>3 cm) lesions
  - Near-complete occlusion
  - Calcific lesions

- Carotid Duplex findings:
  - If peak systolic velocity in the internal carotid artery (ICA) is <125 cm/s, there is mild (<50%) stenosis
  - If peak systolic velocity in the ICA is >230 cm/s, there is severe >70% stenosis. Additional criteria include ICA/common carotid artery (CCA) peak systolic velocity (PSV) ratio >4 and ICA EDV >100 cm/s.
- For patients with carotid stenosis of ≥70% and/or for symptomatic patients with carotid stenosis of 50% to 69%, consider surgical intervention to decrease future risk of stroke. Of note, there are no large prospective randomized outcome studies for these recommendations in the modern era of more aggressive medical therapy with high-dose statins and antiplatelet therapy.
- Risk of stroke with carotid endarterectomy (CEA) in symptomatic patients is higher (<~6%) compared to asymptomatic patients (<~3%)
- Carotid artery stenting compared to CEA is associated with less periprocedural myocardial infarction but possibly higher risk of stroke (especially when performed with operators with more limited experience)
- Some indications to consider for carotid artery stenting (rather than CEA):
  - High-risk CEA candidate
  - History of damage to the contralateral vocal cord
  - Previous neck surgery on the ipsilateral side
  - Neck irradiation
  - Restenosis after CEA
- Approximate risk of combined CABG and carotid surgery:
  - 3% to 4% risk of stroke in staged approach
  - 2% to 3% risk of stroke in simultaneous approach
  - 14% risk of stroke if CABG first and then carotid endarterectomy
- Aspirin decreases the risk of stroke by ~25% in patients with carotid artery disease
- Aorto-ostial carotid lesions → treat with balloon expandable stent
- Carotid bifurcation lesions → treat with self-expanding stent
- Cerebral arteries have no external elastic lamina
- Vertebral artery peak systolic velocity is 20 to 60 cm/s; if >108 cm/s, there is likely a stenosis

- If a patient presents with dizziness, blurred vision, and gait instability, consider vertebral insufficiency

ADDITIONAL CONDITIONS IN PERIPHERAL VASCULAR DISEASE

- Renal artery stenosis (RAS) screening (class I indications):
  - Onset of hypertension before the age of 30 years or severe hypertension after age 55 years
  - Accelerated, resistant, or malignant hypertension
  - Development of new azotemia or worsening renal function after administration of an ACE inhibitor or angiotensin receptor blocker (consider bilateral RAS)
  - Unexplained atrophic kidney or size discrepancy >1.5 cm between kidneys
  - Sudden, unexplained pulmonary edema
- Renal artery intervention with angioplasty/stenting is controversial. Consider for patients with recurrent pulmonary edema when all other causes have been ruled out and significant bilateral renal artery stenosis is present. Can also consider for refractory HTN (on at least 3 medications at optimal doses with one being a diuretic) and worsening renal function in the absence of other causes.
- There is often no family history of HTN in patients with fibromuscular dysplasia; in these patients, balloon angioplasty of the renal artery lesions works well and there is no need for stenting
- Raynaud phenomenon: Redness and pain in extremities to diagnose, can consider checking inflammatory markers (CRP, erythrocyte sedimentation rate [ESR]) and perform nailfold capillaroscopy
  - 1° Raynaud: Female; <40 years old; bilateral; toes involved; no ischemic changes
  - 2° Raynaud: Male; >40 years old; usually unilateral; toes not involved; +ischemic changes
- Mycotic infected pseudoaneurysm → best therapy is to operate (antibiotics likely not adequate)
- Femoral pseudoaneurysms of ≤2 cm can be observed

- Popliteal aneurysm: ~50% bilateral and ~40% have aneurysms in other vascular regions
- Artery of Adamkiewicz arises in T8 to T12 left side ~75% of the time
- Chronic pernio:
  - More common in females
  - Blueness to toes in autumn
  - Vasospastic disease with history of cold injury
- Most common variant of the aortic arch is a common origin of the innominate artery and the left common carotid artery
- Lipedema:
  - Always bilateral
  - Toes not involved
  - Treat with compression stocking
  - Diuretic not helpful
- Lymphedema:
  - More common in women
  - <40 years old
  - ~50% bilateral
  - Painless
  - Toes involved
  - Thick skin
  - Treat with compression stocking (not diuretic)
  - Not much improvement after sleeping
  - Consider lymphoscintigram for diagnosis
- May-Thurner syndrome → left iliac vein is compressed by the right common iliac artery
- Erythromelalgia → rare condition of burning pain, warmth, and redness of the extremities. Etiology is mostly unknown but some conditions to keep in mind:
  - Myeloproliferative disorders (eg, polycythemia vera or essential thrombocytosis)
  - Medications (eg, bromocriptine, calcium channel blockers)
  - Infection (HIV)
  - Mushroom poisoning
  - Diabetes
  - SLE
  - Gout
  - Rheumatoid arthritis

15 Echocardiography

- Structures in the right atrium not to be confused for abnormal masses include:
  - Chiari network
  - Eustachian valve
- Normally, the tricuspid valve is lower than the mitral valve
- Position of AV cusps on TTE:
  - In the parasternal long view, the right and noncoronary cusps are visible. The noncoronary cusp in this view is the inferior one near the left atrium. The left coronary cusp is not visualized.
  - In the short-axis view, the noncoronary cusp is at the intersection of the atrial septum as shown in Figure 15.1.

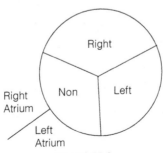

Figure 15.1

- Position of the AV cusps on TEE: noncoronary cusp is at the intersection of the atrial septum (Figure 15.2).

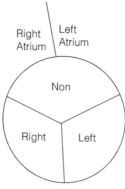

Figure 15.2

- A rare complication of transesophageal echocardiography to keep in mind is pneumohydropericardium
- Grading of aortic atherosclerotic plaque on echocardiography:
  - Grade 1: mild irregularities
  - Grade 2: plaques <3 mm
  - Grade 3: plaques >3 mm
  - Grade 4: protruding plaque
- Modified Bernoulli's equation:
  - $P = 4\ V^2$
    - where P = pressure; V = velocity
- Pressure halftime (PHT) = DT × 0.29 (where DT is the deceleration time)
- Mitral valve area (MVA) = 220/PHT
- Tricuspid valve area (TVA) = 190/PHT
- Flow = velocity × area
- $(V \times A)_{LVOT} = (V \times A)_{Aortic\ Valve}$

- $$AVA = \frac{(LVOT\ diameter)^2 \times 0.785 \times TVI(LVOT)}{TVI(AV)}$$

  - where AVA = AV area; TVI = time volume integral

- If $\dfrac{TVI\ LVOT}{TVI\ AV} < 0.25$, the aortic stenosis is severe

- $SV = CSA \times TVI$
  - where SV = stroke volume; CSA = cross-sectional area; TVI = time volume integral
- $CSA = \pi r^2 = D^2 \times \pi/4 = D^2 \times 0.78$
  - where r = radius; D = diameter; $\pi = 3.14$
- Severe aortic regurgitation → DT is <250 ms
- Calculation of regurgitant fraction for aortic regurgitation: RF = (AoSV–PSV)/AoSV
  - where RF = regurgitant fraction; AoSV = aortic stroke volume; PSV = pulmonic stroke volume
- Calculation of regurgitant fraction for mitral regurgitation: RF = (MSV–Aortic SV)/MSV
  - where RF = regurgitant fraction; MSV = mitral stroke volume; Aortic SV = aortic stroke volume
- (Mitral valve stroke volume) – (LVOT stroke volume) = mitral regurgitation volume
- Regurgitant Fraction (RF) $= \dfrac{(TV - CO/HR)}{Total\ Volume}$

  $= \dfrac{Regurgitant\ Volume\ (RV)}{Total\ Volume}$
  - where TV = total volume; forward volume = CO/HR
- IVC imaging by TTE:
  - Normal IVC <1.7 cm
  - Normal IVC size with 50% collapse of IVC correlates with RA pressure of 0 to 5 mm Hg
  - IVC of >1.7 cm with 50% collapse of IVC correlates with RA pressure of 6 to 10 mm Hg
  - IVC >1.7 cm with <50% collapse of IVC correlates with RA pressure of 10 to 15 mm Hg
  - IVC >1.7 cm with no collapse of IVC correlates with RA pressure of >15 mm Hg
- Tricuspid annular plane systolic excursion (TAPSE) ≤18 mm is abnormal
- Normal LVOT velocity time integral (VTI) → 18 to 22 cm
- Persistence of diastolic flow, consider:
  - Coarctation of the aorta
  - PDA
- Left atrial velocity <20 cm/s increases risk of emboli; >80% to 90% of clots form in the left atrial appendage

- Normal E' ≥10 cm/s (young patients) and ≥8 cm/s (middle-age/elderly patients)
- Pulmonary arterial wedge pressure = 1.9 + 1.24 × E/E'
- E/E' <8 → normal
- E/E' >15 → elevated LVEDP
- Deceleration time in restrictive CMP <160 ms
- Normal tissue Doppler S' >12 to 15 cm/s
- Mitral annular velocity with tissue Doppler is elevated with constriction (>20 cm/s is severe)
- RVOT Doppler pattern:

  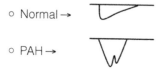

  - Normal →
  - PAH →

- In asymptomatic valvular stenotic patients, follow-up echocardiogram is recommended as follows:
  - Mild → repeat TTE in 3 to 5 years
  - Moderate → repeat TTE in 1 to 2 years
  - Severe → repeat TTE in 6 to 12 months
- SVC velocities with COPD show respirophasic exaggerated variation, whereas in constriction, this is blunted
- Mitral annular velocity in constriction:
  - Lateral wall velocities are less than medial wall velocities
  - E' is high with constriction
- Right ventricular systolic pressure can be calculated in the presence of a VSD and in the absence of any aortic valvular lesions using the systemic blood pressure (this assumes LVSP is equal to the systemic systolic blood pressure) as follows:
  - $RVSP = LVSP - 4\,(VSD)^2$
    - where RVSP = right ventricular systolic pressure; LVSP = left ventricular systolic pressure; VSD = ventricular septal gradient
- $RVSP = 4(V_{TR})^2 + RAP$
  - where V_{TR} = tricuspid valve velocity; RAP = RA pressure

- $PADP = 4(V_{ePR})^2 + RAP$
  - where PADP = PA diastolic pressure
- $PAP_m = TVI_{TR} + RAP$
  - where mean PA pressure; TVI = time-velocity integral
- Modified Quinones equation for calculation of LVEF:
  - $\rightarrow LVEF = ((LVEDD)^2 - (LVESD)^2) / (LVEDD)^2$
    - where LVEDD = left ventricular end-diastolic dimension (mm); LVESD = left ventricular end-systolic dimension (mm)
- Area of the orifice = regurgitant flow/velocity through the orifice
- $ERO = ((2\ \pi r^2) \times (V\ aliasing))/Vmax$
  - where ERO = effective regurgitant orifice
- Mitral valve ERO = (MR volume)/(MR TVI)

- LV index of myocardial performance
$$= \frac{\text{Mitral valve closure to opening} - (ET)}{(ET)}$$

  - where ET = ejection time

16 Interventional Cardiology

- Definition of the waves on atrial tracing:
  - "v"-wave—Atrial "venous" or passive filling
  - "a"-wave—Atrial contraction
  - "c"-wave—Closure and protrusion of the tricuspid valve into the right atrium
  - "x"-descent—Relaxation of RA (pulling of tricuspid annulus downward by RV contraction)
  - "y"-descent—tricuspid valve (TV) opening and RA emptying into RV
- Examples of common abnormalities in RA filling:
  - Increased "a"-wave
    - Tricuspid stenosis
    - Right heart failure
    - Decreased RV compliance
    - Pulmonary HTN
  - Cannon "a"-wave
    - Atria contracting against closed TV (ie, VT, third-degree atrio-ventricular block [AVB])
  - Absent "a"-wave
    - Atrial flutter or fibrillation
  - Elevated "v"-wave
    - Tricuspid regurgitation
  - Prominent "y"-descent
    - Tricuspid regurgitation
  - Prominent "x"- and "y"-descents
    - Constriction/restriction
  - Slow "y"-descent
    - Tricuspid stenosis
    - Tamponade

Table 16.1 Coronary artery lesion classification Characteristics

Type A	• Discrete (<10 mm)
	• Little or no calcium
	• Not ostial or at bifurcation
	• Not tortuous
Type B	• Tubular 10–20 mm
	• Eccentric
	• Moderate tortuosity/angulation
	• Moderate/heavy calcification
	• Ostial
	• Bifurcating lesion
	• Thrombotic
	• Total occlusion (<3 months)
Type C	• Diffuse ≥ 20 mm
	• Very tortuous
	• Very calcific
	• Total occlusion (>3 months)
	• Degenerated old vein grafts

Source: Ryan, Faxon, Gunnar, et al. 1988; Krone, Laskey, Johnson, et al. 2000.

- Risk of emergent CABG for PCI is ~0.4%
- Some PCI complications to keep in mind:
  o Bleeding/retroperitoneal bleed
  o Vascular trauma (peripheral/aortic/coronary)
  o Periprocedure MI
  o Contrast-induced nephropathy
  o Cholesterol/atheroembolization
  o Stent thrombosis
  o Arrhythmias

Essential Facts: Cholesterol/Atheroembolization
- May present with worsening renal function and increasing creatinine
- Blue/gangrene toes
- Livido retivularis may be present
- Eosinophilia may be present
- Histology shows intravascular cholesterol crystals

- Duration of DAPT therapy after PCI continues to be controversial. As it stands now:
  - For elective bare metal stent → 1 month of DAPT then daily aspirin chronically
  - For elective drug-eluting stent → 6 months of DAPT then daily aspirin chronically (some patients with high ischemic risk DAPT duration can be extended, and for other patients with high bleeding risk, a shorter duration of 3 months of DAPT can be considered)
  - For ACS patients, bare metal stent (BMS) or drug eluting stent (DES) → DAPT for 12 months then daily aspirin chronically
- Size of coronary stent should be 1:1 with the reference lumen; intravascular ultrasound (IVUS) and optical coherence tomography (OCT) very helpful in size assessment
- There is no class I indication for IVUS at this time
- Common femoral pseudoaneurysm of ≤2 cm can be observed; ~90% of these thrombose at ~3 weeks
- Bezold-Jarisch reflex can result in abnormal respiration and bradycardia
  - Treat with atropine and phenylephrine
- Endothelial dependent vasodilators:
  - Bradykinin
  - Acetylcholine
- Endothelial independent vasodilators:
  - Nitroglycerine
  - Nipride
- Acetylcholine → impacts endothelium, epicardial arteries, and microcirculation
- Adenosine → impacts microcirculation
- Nitroglycerin/nitric oxide increase cGMP (not cAMP) levels in smooth muscle cells
- Pulmonary artery catheterization:
  - PA line-guided therapy has not been shown to improve survival or change rate of hospitalization
  - Risk of RBBB with right heart catheterization is ~3% to 10%
  - Risk of complete heart block with right heart catheterization in a patient with underlying LBBB is very

low—there is no requirement for placement of a temporary wire for such cases, but standby external pacemakers and equipment for transvenous pacemaker insertion should be readily available

- Syntax score:
  - Low score (0–22) → CABG vs PCI no difference in terms of survival
  - Intermediate score (23–32) → CABG vs PCI no difference in terms of survival
  - High score (> 32) → CABG is superior to multivessel PCI in terms of 2-year survival (Serruys, Morice, Kappetein, et al. 2009)
- CABG is generally the more preferred option for revascularization in patients with multivessel CAD (including proximal LAD or left main), especially in diabetes, low ejection fraction (EF), poor compliant patients, high Syntax score
- Note that in chronic stable angina, elective PCI is performed mainly for symptomatic relief, but for left main and high-grade proximal LAD, there is also survival benefit with revascularization
- In general, CABG vs PCI for multivessel CAD:
  - Associated with similar survival (per the Syntax scores outlined)
  - Increased risk of stroke with CABG
  - Need for further procedures is more with PCI
  - Longer recovery time with CABG
  - Monotherapy with an antiplatelet agent after CABG as opposed to DAPT after PCI
- PCI should not be performed in patients who are not compliant with medications
- Resolution of IVUS is ~150 μm vs resolution of OCT, which is ~10 μm
- On IVUS, to identify the true lumen vs false lumen, look for:
  - Trilaminar appearance
  - Presence of side branches
- IVUS-guided PCI:
  - Results in larger acute lumen gain
  - Less angiographic restenosis

- ○ Less repeat revascularization
- ○ But no change in risk of future myocardial infarction
- Clopidogrel (Plavix) load of 600 mg results in maximal platelet inhibition in ~2 hours
- Clopidogrel inhibits ADP P2Y12 and increases cAMP and VASP-P (vasodilator-stimulated phosphoprotein)
- Clopidogrel poor metabolizer are ~3% whites, ~5% African Americans, ~15% Asians
  - ○ CYP2C19 polymorphism accounts for only ~12% of the % variability in platelet responsiveness to Plavix
  - ○ Poor metabolizers are *2/*2
  - ○ Ultra-rapid metabolizers are *1/*17 and *17/*17
- Triple therapy with aspirin, clopidogrel, and warfarin is associated with ~2.2% risk of major bleeding at 30 days
- Medina classification nomenclature for bifurcation lesions refers to the vessels in the following order → proximal/distal/side branch
- During pulmonary valvuloplasty, if the patient becomes hypotensive, avoid using dopamine or epinephrine as the subvalvular obstruction will get worse
- Slope of the end-systolic pressure-volume relation (ESPVR) shifts to the left with increased contractility
- Alcohol ablation and septal myomectomy → similar mortality
- Mitral stenosis valvuloplasty indications:
  - ○ MVA ≤1.5 cm^2
  - ○ Wilkin's score of ≤8
  - ○ PA pressure of >50 mm Hg at rest or >60 mm Hg with exercise
- Wilkin's score for assessment of mitral valvuloplasty includes the following (each is graded from 1 [normal] to 4 [very abnormal]). Best outcomes with balloon valvuloplasty are achieved if score is ≤8.
  - ○ Leaflet mobility
  - ○ Valve thickening
  - ○ Calcification
  - ○ Subvalvular thickening
- After mitral valvuloplasty for mitral stenosis, consider repeating TTE in 1 week. Of note, there is no role for mitral valvuloplasty for a prosthetic valve stenosis.

- Valvuloplasty has no role for mitral stenosis due to prosthetic valve stenosis

---

Essential Facts: Fame Trial
- If FFR >0.8, the 2-year incidence of MI is ~1.8%
- If angiogram showed 50% to 70% stenosis → FFR was negative in ~65%
- If angiogram showed 71% to 90% stenosis → FFR was negative in ~20%
- If angiogram showed ≥90% stenosis → FFR was negative in ~4%

- 2-year major adverse cardiovascular event (MACE) if coronary stenosis is fractional flow reserve (FFR) negative is ~4%
- If adenosine cannot be used for FFR evaluation, consider using intracoronary nitroprusside (100 µg) bolus
- Newer technologies for coronary artery stenosis assessment include iFR (instant wave-free ratio) and non-invasive FFR-CT (which is a noninvasive calculation of FFR based on conventional coronary CT angiography). These technologies are likely to play a more prominent role in the cardiac catheterization laboratory over the upcoming years to assess hemodynamic significance of coronary artery stenoses. A few pointers to keep in mind:
  - iFR is measured at rest without the need to administer pharmacologic agents
  - iFr still requires to pass a wire distal to the coronary stenosis for evaluation normal iFR value is 1.0; below 0.9 it is suggestive of flow restriction
- Abnormal CFR value is <2.0 (can use adenosine, papaverine, dipyridamole for CFR measurement but not acetylcholine)
- Plaque erosion is more common in smoker females
- Vulnerable plaques appear yellow and stable plaques appear white on angioscopy

- Smooth muscle cell proliferation (as seen in in-stent restenosis) is due to increased production of collagen III
- Restenosis definition:
  - Late loss ≥0.7 mm
  - Loss of >50% of acute gain in follow-up imaging
  - Diameter stenosis of >50% at follow-up imaging
- Kugel's artery is a right-to-right collateral in the right coronary artery
- Vieussens' ring includes collaterals from RCA conus to the left system (usually LAD)
- Vieussens' valve is located at the junction of the great cardiac vein and the coronary sinus
- The sinus nodal artery originates from the right coronary artery ~60% of the time and from the left circumflex artery ~40% of the time
- Most common coronary anomaly is the left circumflex artery coming off the RCA and coursing posterior to the aorta
- Posterior mitral papillary muscle is supplied by PDA only, whereas the anterior papillary muscle is supplied by diagonal and obtuse marginal branches
- Severity of valvular regurgitation angiographically (Table 16.2)

Table 16.2 Grading of valvular regurgitation severity angiographically

Grade I	Partial filling of the chamber regurgitant contrast enters
Grade II	Chamber regurgitant contrast enters is less dense than the chamber being injected into
Grade III	Chamber regurgitant contrast enters is same density as chamber being injected into with 4–5 heartbeats
Grade IV	Chamber regurgitant contrast enters is same density as chamber being injected into with <3 heartbeats

Source: Grossman 2000; Otto 2004.

- Blush score:
  - 0 = no blush
  - 1 = contrast persistent stain
  - 2 = contrast dissipates slowly
  - 3 = normal
- Coronary artery dissections (Table 16.3)

Table 16.3 Classification of coronary artery dissections

Type	Description	Risk of Acute Closure
Type A	Mild luminal haziness almost	0%
Type B	Intraluminal abnormality	~3%
Type C	Extraluminal abnormality/dye	~10%
Type D	Spiral dissection	~30%
Type E	Dissection with filling defects	~10%
Type F	Dissection with poor/limited distal flow	~70%

Source: Rogers, Lasala 2004; Eshtehardi, Adorjan, Togni 2010.

- Risk factors for spontaneous coronary artery dissection:
  - Advanced maternal age
  - Third trimester of pregnancy
  - Multigravida
- Coronary artery perforations:
  - Type I—extraluminal contrast noted but no extravasation
  - Type II—epicardial/myocardial blush but no extravasation
  - Type III—extravasation (IIIA toward pericardium; IIIB toward myocardium)
- Bleeding Academic Research Consortium definition (Table 16.4)
- Retroperitoneal bleed can be associated with a high mortality if not recognized and treated emergently. The incidence is ~0.7%. Risk factors for retroperitoneal bleed include:
  - High femoral puncture site
  - Female
  - BSA of <1.7 m^2

Table 16.4 BARC Definition for bleeding

Type 0	No bleed
Type I	Minor
Type II	Any overt, actionable sign of hemorrhage
Type III	
a.	↓ 3–5 g/dL Hgb
b.	↓ >5 g/dL Hgb
c.	Intracranial/intra-occular bleed
Type IV	CABG bleed
Type V	Fatal

Source: Mehran, Rao, Bhatt, et al. 2011.

- Chronic total occlusions → more complex crossing them if no beak, lots of bridging collaterals are present, at a side branch, old lesion, long lesion
- Saphenous vein graft (SVG) disease:
  ○ Subacute thrombosis (usually <1 month after CABG)
  ○ Neointimal hyperplasia (1 month to 1 year)
  ○ Atheroscleross (usually >3 years after CABG)
- There is a ~25% chance of graft occlusion at 1 year if the coronary artery that is bypassed has <50% stenosis
- Predictors of Saphenous vein graft failure:
  ○ Young patient age
  ○ LVEF <30%
  ○ Older age graft
  ○ Large conduit diameter
  ○ Endoscopic vein harvest
  ○ Smaller target artery diameter
- Embolic devices for the treatment of SVG disease decrease the risk of MI but not death or emergency bypass
- PCI of SVG with covered stent has worse outcome than with bare metal stent
- To shorten a guide catheter, use a piece of sheath one size *smaller*
- Sheath sizes reflect internal diameter, whereas guide catheters reflect external diameters

- Late loss index after angioplasty is calculated as:
  - Late loss index = (late loss)/(acute gain)
- If there is a pulmonary artery perforation, turn the patient to the side of the perforation to avoid issues with the good side
- Acute cortical blindness can be associated with a large contrast dose exposure
- Categories of contrast agents with some examples:
  - Hyperosmolar (Hypaque—ionic contrast)
  - Isoosmolar (iodixanol [Visipaque]—nonionic contrast)
  - Low osmolar (iohexol [Omnipaque]—nonionic contrast; ioxaglate [Hexabrix]—ionic contrast)
- Allergic contrast reaction occurs likely from activation of direct complement and degranulation of mast cells and basophils
- Contrast reaction should be treated as:
  - Moderate reaction: 0.3 to 0.5 mL (0.3–0.5mg) of 1:1000 epinephrine (EPI) given IM or SC
  - Severe reaction: 1 mL (0.1 mg) of 1:10,000 EPI given IV (can repeat if no improvement in ~10–15 minutes)
    - Also consider IV hydration, steroids, dopamine, Benadryl therapy
- Cross-reaction between ionic and nonionic contrast is very low (<1%)
- Formula to estimate approximate contrast volume use in a case: ~3.7 × estimated glomerular filtration rate (eGFR)
- Best ways of reducing contrast induced nephropathy (CIN):
  - Limit contrast use
  - Hydration pre/post
  - Avoiding other nephrotoxic agents periprocedurally
- Asymptomatic increase in the creatinine kinase (CK) level (>5 times upper limit of normal) can occur in up to 3% to 10% of successful PCI cases
- Presence of chronic total occlusion (CTO) in a non-infarct-related artery is a strong independent predictor of increased 5-year mortality

Table 16.5. Contrast-induced nephropathy risk score

Risk Factor	Points
Hypotension	5 points
IABP	5 points
CHF	5 points
Age ≥75	4 points
Anemia	3 points
Diabetes	3 points
GFR <60 or serum creatinine >1.5	2–6 points
Contrast amount	1 point for each 100 mL contrast used

Score	Risk of CIN	Risk of hemodialysis
≤5	7.5%	0%–0.4%
6–10	14%	0.12%
11–16	26%	1.1%
≥16	57%	12%

Source: Mehran, Aymong, Nikolsky, et al. 2004.

- Risk of bleeding increases with:
  - Increasing age
  - Female sex
  - Renal insufficiency
  - Low weight
- If performing PCI on Lovenox and the patient last received a dose >8 hours prior, give a dose of 0.3 mg/kg IV×1

Essential Facts: Brachytherapy
- Recurrent Instent restenosis (ISR) is >20%
- Most restenosis after brachytherapy happens <6 months

- Stent fracture:
  - Appears to be more common in the mid-RCA location
  - Overall, ~3% to 4% risk
  - Also, longer stents, stent overexpansion, and overlapping stents are risk factors for stent fracture
- Predictors of mortality at 1 year after PCI:
  - Older age (>70 years)
  - Tachyarrhythmias
  - Weight <80 kg
  - Number of vessels with coronary artery disease
  - LVEF (odds ratio increases 1.5 with every 10% decrease in LVEF)

RADIATION

- Roentgen (R) = intensity of x-ray exposure
- Gray (Gy) = absorption of energy → good for monitoring of skin injury
- Sievert (Sv) = measure of whole-body biologic effect → good for monitoring long-term risk of cancer
- Accepted yearly radiation dose is ~50 mSv
- Background normal radiation is ~3 to 4 mSv/y
- 10 mSv → about 500 chest x-ray or ~3 years of natural background radiation exposure
- Dose area product (DAP) is the total x-ray energy detected during the procedure, and it reflects the total amount of radiation. It is calculated by:
  - DAP = KERMA × CSA
    - Where KERMA is kinetic energy released to matter and CSA is cross-sectional area
- Collimation will do the following:
  - Decrease beam area
  - Decrease DAP
  - Decrease total patient dose
  - Decrease room exposure
  - Does not reduce the skin entrance dose to the patient
- In pregnant patients, external shielding is likely not very helpful to the fetus as this does not block the internal scatter radiation.

- Factors that increase entry dose to the patient:
  - Obese patient
  - Long x-ray/imaging duration
  - Angulated/steep views
  - High-intensity mode and high image magnification
  - Defective/old x-ray machine
- Effects of radiation:
  - Stochastic
    - Effects that occur by chance (eg, cancer and genetic effects)
    - There is no threshold dose but risk increases with dose
  - Nonstochastic (otherwise known as deterministic effects)—these effects are more dose dependent:
    - Skin: Erythema (~2 Gy exposure: within hours); hair loss (~3–7 Gy: in ~3–4 weeks); desquamation of skin (~8–14 Gy: in ~4 weeks); dermal atrophy/necrosis (~10–12 Gy: months to year); telangiectasia (~10 Gy: in ~12 months)
    - Cataracts
    - Sterility
    - GI side effects
    - CNS side effects
    - Hematologic effects
- Radiation side effects on the heart:
  - Can result in premature coronary artery disease, cardiomyopathy, pericardial disease, and valvulopathy
  - Usually impact is 10 to 15 years after radiation exposure to the heart
  - Regurgitant valvular lesions are more common than stenosis but aortic stenosis can occur

17 Cardiac Tumors

- Primary cardiac tumors are rare (<1% of all cardiac tumors) and most are metastatic tumors to the heart
- Primary cardiac tumors:
  - Benign—some examples include:
    - Myxoma—most common
    - Papillary fibroelastoma—second most common
    - Lipoma
    - Rhabdomyoma—most common in infants/children
    - Hemangioma
    - Fibroma
  - Malignant—some examples include:
    - Sarcomas—rhabdomyosarcoma, angiosarcoma, fibrosarcoma, leiomyosarcoma
    - Teratoma
    - Mesothelioma
- Secondary (metastatic cardiac tumors)—some of the more common ones that might metastasize to the heart/pericardium:
  - Thyroid
  - Lung
  - Breast
  - Esophagus
  - Kidney
  - Lymphoma
  - Leukemia
  - Melanoma
- Most common cardiac tumors in adults: myxoma, fibroelastoma, rhabdomyoma

- Most common cardiac tumors in kids: rhabdomyoma (most common), fibroma, sarcoma
- Most common pericardial tumor in adults: mesothelioma
- Most common pericardial tumor in infants: teratoma
- Tuberous sclerosis:
  - Autosomal dominant
  - Association with seizures
  - Association with mental developmental delay
  - Association with facial angiofibromas
  - Rhabdomyoma
- Atrial myxoma:
  - More common in the left >> right atrium
  - Mitral regurgitation is the most common murmur with patients with left atrial myxoma
  - If very large, mitral stenosis–like clinical presentation and a tumor plop can be audible
  - Systemic embolization in about 25% of patients
  - More common in women
  - Constitutional symptoms of fevers/weight loss in ~30%
  - After respective surgery, recurrence rate can be ~2% to 5%
  - Cardiac myxomas have been associated with Cushing syndrome
- Carney complex:
  - Autosomal dominant
  - Cardiac myxoma and other myxomas
  - Pigmentation abnormalities such as lentigines and blue nevi on the face, neck, and trunk
  - Possible pituitary adenomas; ↑ growth hormone and acromegaly
  - Associated with breast ductal adenoma and possibly testicular tumors
- Papillary fibroelastoma:
  - More common on left-sided cardiac valves
  - Can result in systemic embolization
  - Often incidentally note on echocardiography
  - Treatment:

- - Surgical, especially in patients with history of systemic embolization
  - Recurrence after surgical resection unlikely
  - For right-sided valvular fibroelastoma, one can possibly consider nonoperative approach and observation if the lesion is not growing
  - Anticoagulation is controversial
- Lambl's excrescences (small filiform processes) most common on the aortic valve (more so than on the mitral valve)
- Libman-Sachs endocarditis:
  - Nonbacterial endocarditis can be seen with SLE and APLS
  - More common on the mitral valve
  - Rarely results in systemic embolization
  - If associated with malignancy, the risk of embolization is higher

18 Formulas

Table 18.1 Abbreviations used in these equations

CO = cardiac output
DBP = diastolic blood pressure
DEP = diastolic ejection period
EDV = end diastolic volume
ESV = end systolic volume
FA = femoral (or any) artery
Hgb = hemoglobin
HR = heart rate
PA = pulmonary artery
PV = pulmonary vein
Qp = pulmonic flow
Qs = systemic flow
SBP = systolic blood pressure
SEP = systolic ejection period
SV = stroke volume

- Wall stress (La Place equation) = Pressure × (radius)^2/thickness
- Mean arterial pressure = (SBP + (DBP × 2))/3
- CO = HR × SV
- PVR = ((PA − PCWP)/pulmonary blood flow)
  - Woods units × 80 = Dynes-s/cm^5
- SVR = (mean arterial pressure − mean RA pressure)/systemic blood flow
- Creatinine clearance = (140 − age)(wt in kg)(0.85 for females)/72 × creatinine

Table 18.2 "Rule of 6s"

Mean right atrial pressure	6 mm Hg
Right ventricular pressure	24/6 mm Hg
Pulmonary artery pressure	24/12 mm Hg
Pulmonary capillary wedge pressure	12 mm Hg

Note: All numbers are divisible by 6 to estimate normal average cardiac filling pressures.

- Mixed venous saturation:
  - $MVO_2 = (3SVC + 1IVC)/4$
- Calculation of cardiac output:
  - $CO = (VO_2)/(1.34) \times (Hgb) \times (FA - PA\%)$
    - VO_2 is oxygen consumption
- Calculation of pulmonary blood flow (PBF)
  - $\rightarrow PBF = O_2$ consumption/(10) (1.36) (Hgb) $(PV - PAO_2$ difference)
- Calculation of systemic blood flow (SBF)
  - $SBF = O_2$ consumption/(10) (1.36) (Hgb) $(PA - MVO_2$ difference), or
  - $SBF \times (Qp/Qs) = PBF$
- Calculation of effective blood flow (EBF)
  - $EBF = O_2$ consumption/(10) (1.36) (Hgb) $(PV - MVO_2$ difference)
- Shunt calculation:
  - $Qp/Qs = (arterial - MVO_2)/(PV - PAO_2)$
- Another way of calculating shunt:
  - Left-to-right shunt $= PBF - EBF = PBF - SBF$ (assuming $EBF = SBF$)
  - Right-to-left shunt $= SBF - EBF$
- Calculation of aortic valve area (Gorlin formula):
  - $AVA =$ Valve flow (cc/s)$/K \times C \times \sqrt{}$ aortic valve gradient
    - $K = 44.3$; $C = 1$ for AV
- Valve flow $=$ CO (cc/min)/SEP (s/min) $=$ CO/SEP (s/beat) $\times$ HR
- Hakki formula (for aortic valve area calculation):
  - $AVA = CO/\sqrt{}$ aortic valve gradient
- Calculation of mitral valve area:
  - $MVA =$ Valve flow (cc/s)$/K \times C \times \sqrt{}$ gradient
    - $K = 44.3$; $C = 0.85$ for MV

- Valve flow = CO (cc/min)/DEP (s/min) = CO/DEP (s/beat) × HR
- Left ventricular ejection fraction (LVEF)
  - LVEF = EDV − ESV/EDV, or
  - LVEF = SV/EDV
- Cardiac power = (MAP × CO)/451
  - Best predictor of mortality in shock
- Approximate formula to convert JVP on exam to pressure in mm Hg:
  - JVP (in cm) × 0.7 = pressure in mm Hg (in the RA)

References

ACCF/SCAI Premier Interventional Cardiology Overview and Board Preparatory Course, August 17–19, 2012. Dallas, TX: The Ritz-Carlton; 2012.

Amsterdam EA, Wenger NK, Brindis RG, et al. 2014 AHA/ACC guideline for the management of patients with non-ST-elevation acute coronary syndromes: executive summary: a report of the American College of Cardiology/American Heart Association Task Force on Practice Guidelines. *Circulation.* 2014;130:2354.

Anderson JL, Halperin JL, Albert NM, et al. Management of patients with peripheral artery disease (compilation of 2005 and 2011 ACCF/AHA guideline recommendations): a report of the American College of Cardiology Foundation/American Heart Association Task Force on Practice Guidelines. *J Am Coll Cardiol.* 2013;61:1555–1570.

Arger PH, Iyoob SD. *The Complete Guide to Vascular Ultrasound.* Philadelphia, PA: Lippincott Williams & Wilkins; 2004.

Baim DS, Grossman W. *Cardiac Catheterization, Angiography, and Intervention.* 6th ed. Philadelphia, PA: Lippincott Williams & Wilkins; 2000.

Baliga RR, ed. *McGraw-Hill Specialty Board Review—Cardiology.* New York, NY: McGraw-Hill Medical; 2012.

Bonaca MP, Lewis GD, O'Donoghue ML, Tedrow UB. *Pocket Notebook—Pocket Cardiology—A Companion to Pocket Medicine.* Philadelphia, PA: Wolters Kluwer; 2016.

Brott TG, Halperin JL, Abbara S, et al. 2011 ASA/ACCF/AHA/AANN/AANS/ACR/ASNR/CNS/SAIP/SCAI/SIR/SNIS/SVM/SVS guideline on the management of patients with extracranial carotid and vertebral artery disease: a report of the American College of Cardiology Foundation/American Heart Association Task Force on Practice Guidelines, and the American Stroke Association, American Association of

Neuroscience Nurses, American Association of Neurological Surgeons, American College of Radiology, American Society of Neuroradiology, Congress of Neurological Surgeons, Society of Atherosclerosis Imaging and Prevention, Society for Cardiovascular Angiography and Interventions, Society of Interventional Radiology, Society of NeuroInterventional Surgery, Society for Vascular Medicine, and Society for Vascular Surgery developed in collaboration with the American Academy of Neurology and Society of Cardiovascular Computed Tomography. *J Am Coll Cardiol*. 2011;124(4):489–532.

Casserly IP, Schar R, Yadav JS. *Manual of Peripheral Vascular Intervention*. Philadelphia, PA: Lippincott Williams & Wilkins; 2005.

Chou T-C, Knilans TK. *Electrocardiography in Clinical Practice Adult and Pediatrics*. 4th ed. Philadelphia, PA: W. B. Saunders; 1996.

Eckel RH, Jakicic JM, Ard JD, et al. 2013 AHA/ACC guideline on lifestyle management to reduce cardiovascular risk: a report of the American College of Cardiology/American Heart Association Task Force on Practice Guidelines. *Circulation*. 2014;129(25)(suppl 2):S76-S99.

Fihn SD, Gardin JM, Abrams J, et al. 2012 ACCF/AHA/ACP/AATS/PCNA/SCAI/STS guideline for the diagnosis and management of patients with stable ischemic heart disease: a report of the American College of Cardiology Foundation/American Heart Association Task Force on Practice Guidelines, and the American College of Physicians, American Association for Thoracic Surgery, Preventive Cardiovascular Nurses Association, Society for Cardiovascular Angiography and Interventions, and Society of Thoracic Surgeons. *J Am Coll Cardiol*. 2012;126(25):3097–3137.

Fleisher LA, Fleischmann KE, Auerbach AD, et al. 2014 ACC/AHA guideline on perioperative cardiovascular evaluation and management of patients undergoing noncardiac surgery: a report of the American College of Cardiology/American Heart Association Task Force on Practice Guidelines. *J Am Coll Cardiol*. 2014;130(24):2215–2245.

Gerhard-Herman MD, Gornik HL, Barrett C, et al. 2016 AHA/ACC guideline on the management of patients with lower extremity peripheral artery disease: executive summary. A report of the American College of Cardiology/American Heart Association Task Force on Clinical Practice Guidelines. *J Am Coll Cardiol*. [Epub ahead of print]

Gersh BJ, Maron BJ, Bonow RO, et al. 2011 ACCF/AHA guideline for the diagnosis and treatment of hypertrophic cardiomyopathy: a report of the American College of Cardiology Foundation/American Heart Association Task Force on Practice Guidelines developed in Collaboration with the American Association for Thoracic Surgery, American Society of Echocardiography, American Society of Nuclear Cardiology, Heart Failure Society of America, Heart Rhythm Society, Society for Cardiovascular Angiography and Interventions, and Society of Thoracic Surgeons. *J Am Coll Cardiol.* 2011; 58(25):e212-e260.

Goff DC, Lloyd-Jones DM, Bennett G, et al. 2013 ACC/AHA guideline on the assessment of cardiovascular risk: a report of the American College of Cardiology/American Heart Association Task Force on Practice Guidelines. *J Am Coll Cardiol.* 2014;129(25)(suppl 2):S49-S73.

Grines CL, Savu MA, Tejada LA. *Interventional Cardiology: The Essentials for the Board, Questions and Answers, Clinical Cases and Pearls.* Armonk, NY: Futura; 1999.

Harold JG, Bass TA, Bashore TM, et al. ACCF/AHA/SCAI 2013 update of the clinical competence statement on coronary artery interventional procedures: a report of the American College of Cardiology Foundation/American Heart Association/American College of Physicians Task Force on Clinical Competence and Training (Writing Committee to Revise the 2007 Clinical Competence Statement on Cardiac Interventional Procedures). *Circulation.* 2013;128(4):436–472.

Hillis LD, Smith PK, Anderson JL, et al. 2011 ACCF/AHA guideline for coronary artery bypass graft surgery: a report of the American College of Cardiology Foundation/American Heart Association Task Force on Practice Guidelines developed in Collaboration with the American Association for Thoracic Surgery, Society of Cardiovascular Anesthesiologists, and Society of Thoracic Surgeons. *J Am Coll Cardiol.* 2011;58(24):e123-e210.

Hiratzka LF, Creager MA, Isselbacher EM, et al. Surgery for Aortic dilatation in patients with bicuspid aortic valves: a statement of clarification from the American College of Cardiology/American Heart Association Task Force on Clinical Practice Guidelines. *J Am Coll Cardiol.* 2016;133(7):680–686.

Jensen MD, Ryan DH, Apovian CM, et al. 2013 AHA/ACC/TOS guideline for the management of overweight and obesity in adults: a report of the American College of Cardiology/American Heart Association Task Force on Practice Guidelines and The Obesity Society. *Circulation.* 2014;129(25)(suppl 2):S102-S138.

Labovitz AJ, Williams GA. *Doppler Echocardiography: The Quantitative Approach.* 3rd ed. Philadelphia, PA: Williams & Wilkins; 1992.

Leon MB, Safian RD, Reed M. *Interventional Cardiology: Self-Assessment and Review, Volumes I & II.* Birmingham, MI: Physician Press; 2000.

Levine GN, Bates ER, Blankenship JC, et al. 2015 ACC/AHA/SCAI focused update on primary percutaneous coronary intervention for patients with ST-elevation myocardial infarction. An update of the 2011 ACCF/AHA/SCAI guideline for percutaneous coronary intervention and the 2013 ACCF/AHA guideline for the management of ST-elevation myocardial infarction. *J Am Coll Cardiol.* [Epub ahead of print]

Lilly LS, Brown JD, Desai AS, Lakdawal N, Miller AL, Pande AN. *Braunwald's Heart Disease: Review and Assessment.* 8th ed. Philadelphia, PA: Saunders Elsevier; 2006.

Lund LH, Edwards LB, Kucheryavaya AY, et al. The Registry of the International Society for Heart and Lung Transplantation: Thirty-second Official Adult Heart Transplantation Report—2015; focus theme: early graft failure. *J Heart Lung Transplant.* 2015;34:1244.

Mann DL, Zipes DP, Libby P, et al. *Braunwald's Heart Disease: A Textbook of Cardiovascular Medicine.* 10th ed. Philadelphia, PA: Elsevier/Saunders; 2015.

Mehra MR, Canter CE, Hannan MM, et al. The 2016 International Society for Heart Lung Transplantation listing criteria for heart transplantation: a 10-year update. *J Heart Lung Transplant.* 2016;35:1.

Mehra MR, Kobashigawa J, Starling R, et al. Listing criteria for heart transplantation: International Society for Heart and Lung Transplantation guidelines for the care of cardiac transplant candidates—2006. *J Heart Lung Transplant.* 2006;25:1024.

Mosca L, Benjamin EJ, Berra K, et al. Effectiveness-based guidelines for the prevention of cardiovascular disease in women—2011 update: a guideline from the American Heart Association. *Circulation.* 2011;123(11):1243–1262.

Mukherjee D, Cho L, Moliterno DJ. *Interventional Cardiology: 1001 Questions: An Interventional Cardiology Board Review.* Philadelphia, PA: Wolters Kluwer Health/Lippincott Williams & Wilkins; 2012.

Murphy JG, Lloyd MA, eds. *Mayo Clinic Cardiology: Concise Textbook*. 4th ed. New York: Mayo Clinic Scientific Press/Oxford University Press; 2013.

Nishimura RA, Otto CM, Bonow RO, et al. 2014 AHA/ACC guideline for the management of patients with valvular heart disease: a report of the American College of Cardiology/American Heart Association Task Force on Practice Guidelines. *J Am Coll Cardiol*. 2014;63(22):e57.

Nishimura RA, Otto CM, Bonow RO, et al. 2017 AHA/ACC focused update of the 2014 AHA/ACC guideline for the management of patients with valvular heart disease: a report of the American College of Cardiology/American Heart Association Task Force on Clinical Practice Guidelines. *J Am Coll Cardiol*. [Epub ahead of print]

O'Gara PT, Kushner FG, Ascheim DD, et al. 2013 ACCF/AHA guideline for the management of ST-elevation myocardial infarction: a report of the American College of Cardiology Foundation/American Heart Association Task Force on Practice Guidelines. *Circulation* 2013;127(4):e362-e425.

O'Rourke RA, Fuster V, Alexander RW, et al. *HURST'S, The Heart: Manual of Cardiology*. 11th ed. New York, NY: McGraw-Hill Medical Publishing Division; 2005.

Otto CM, Pearlman AS. *Textbook of Clinical Echocardiography*. Philadelphia, PA: W. B. Saunders; 1995.

Owens CD, Yeghiazarians Y. *Handbook of Endovascular Peripheral Interventions*. New York, NY: Springer; 2012.

Page RL, Joglar JA, Caldwell MA, et al. 2015 ACC/AHA/HRS guideline for the management of adult patients with supraventricular tachycardia: a report of the American College of Cardiology/American Heart Association Task Force on Clinical Practice Guidelines and the Heart Rhythm Society. *Heart Rhythm Case Reports*. [Epub ahead of print]

Ragosta M. *Textbook of Clinical Hemodynamics*. Philadelphia, PA: W. B. Saunders/Elsevier; 2008.

Rimmerman CM, Jain AK. *Interactive: Electrocardiography*. 2nd ed. Philadelphia, PA: Lippincott Williams & Wilkins; 2008.

Rooke TW, Hirsch AT, Misra S, et al. Management of patients with peripheral artery disease (compilation of 2005 and 2011 ACCF/AHA Guideline Recommendations): a report of the American College of Cardiology Foundation/American Heart Association Task Force on Practice Guidelines. *J Am Coll Cardiol*. 2013;61(14):1555–1570.

Shen W-K, Sheldon RS, Benditt DG, et al. 2017 ACC/AHA/HRS guideline for the evaluation and management of patients with syncope: executive summary: a report of the American College of Cardiology/American Heart Association Task Force on Clinical Practice Guidelines, and the Heart Rhythm Society. *J Am Coll Cardiol.* [Epub ahead of print]

Simonneau G, Gatzoulis MA, Adatia I, et al. Updated clinical classification of pulmonary hypertension. *J Am Coll Cardiol.* 2013;62(25)(suppl):D34.

Smith SC, Benjamin EJ, Bonow RO, et al. AHA/ACCF Secondary prevention and risk reduction therapy for patients with coronary and other atherosclerotic vascular disease: 2011 update. A guideline from the American Heart Association and American College of Cardiology Foundation endorsed by the World Heart Federation and the Preventive Cardiovascular Nurses Association. *J Am Coll Cardiol.* 2011; 124(22):2458–2473.

Stone NJ, Robinson JG, Lichtenstein AH, et al. 2013 ACC/AHA guideline on the treatment of blood cholesterol to reduce atherosclerotic cardiovascular risk in adults: a report of the American College of Cardiology/American Heart Association Task Force on Practice Guidelines. *J Am Coll Cardiol.* 2014;63(25, pt B):2889–2934.

Tracy CM, Epstein AE, Darbar D, et al. 2012 ACCF/AHA/HRS focused update incorporated into the ACCF/AHA/HRS 2008 guidelines for device-based therapy of cardiac rhythm abnormalities: a report of the American College of Cardiology Foundation/American Heart Association Task Force on Practice Guidelines and the Heart Rhythm Society. *J Am Coll Cardiol.* 2013;61(3):1784–1800.

Varosy PD, Chen LY, Miller AL, et al. Pacing as a treatment for reflex-mediated (vasovagal, situational, or carotid sinus hypersensitivity) syncope: a systematic review for the 2017 ACC/AHA/HRS guideline for the evaluation and management of patients with syncope. A report of the American College of Cardiology/American Heart Association Task Force on Clinical Practice Guidelines and the Heart Rhythm Society. *J Am Coll Cardiol.* [Epub ahead of print]

Warnes CA, Williams RG, Bashore TM, et al. ACC/AHA 2008 guidelines for the management of adults with congenital heart disease: a report of the American College of Cardiology/American Heart Association Task Force on Practice Guidelines (Writing Committee to Develop Guidelines on the Management of Adults With Congenital Heart Disease). Developed in collaboration with the American Society of Echocardiography, Heart Rhythm Society, International Society for Adult Congenital Heart Disease, Society for Cardiovascular Angiography and Interventions, and Society of Thoracic Surgeons. *J Am Coll Cardiol.* 2008;52(23):e143-e263.

Writing Committee Members, Gerhard-Herman MD, Gornik HL, Barrett C, et al. 2016 AHA/ACC guideline on the management of patients with lower extremity peripheral artery disease: executive summary. *Vasc Med.* 2017;22(3):NP1-NP43.

Yancy CW, Jessup M, Bozkurt B, et al. 2013 ACCF/AHA guideline for the management of heart failure: executive summary: a report of the American College of Cardiology Foundation/American Heart Association Task Force on practice guidelines. *Circulation.* 2013;128:1810.

Yancy CW, Jessup M, Bozkurt B, et al. 2016 ACC/AHA/HFSA focused update on new pharmacological therapy for heart failure: an update of the 2013 ACCF/AHA guideline for the management of heart failure: a report of the American College of Cardiology/American Heart Association Task Force on Clinical Practice Guidelines and the Heart Failure Society of America. *Circulation.* 2016;134:e282.

Yancy, CW, Jessup M, Bozkurt B, et al. 2017 ACC/AHA/HFSA focused update of the 2013 ACCF/AHA guideline for the management of heart failure: a report of the American College of Cardiology/American Heart Association Task Force on Clinical Practice Guidelines and the Heart Failure Society of America. *J Am Coll Cardiol.* [Epub ahead of print]

WORKS CITED

Alberti KG, Eckel RH, Grundy SM, et al. Harmonizing the metabolic syndrome: a joint interim statement of the International Diabetes Federation Task Force on Epidemiology and Prevention; National Heart, Lung, and Blood Institute; American Heart Association; World Heart Federation; International Atherosclerosis Society; and International Association for the Study of Obesity. *Circulation.* 2009;120(16):1640–1645.

Antman EM, Cohen M, Bernink PJ, et al. The TIMI risk score for unstable angina/non-ST elevation MI: a method for prognostication and therapeutic decision making. *JAMA.* 2000; 284(7):835.

Campeau L. Grading of angina pectoris. *Circulation.* 1976; 54:5223.

Cutlip DE, Windecker S, Mehran R, et al. Clinical end points in coronary stent trials: a case for standardized definitions. *Circulation.* 2007;115(17):2344.

Durack D, Lukes A, Bright D. New criteria for diagnosis of infective endocarditis: utilization of specific echocardiographic findings. Duke Endocarditis Service. *Am J Med.* 1994;96 (3): 200–209.

Eshtehardi P, Adorjan P, Togni M, et al. Iatrogenic left main coronary artery dissection: incidence, classification, management, and long-term follow-up. *Am. Heart J.* 2010; 159(6):1147–1153.

Fontaine R, Kim M, Kieny R. Surgical treatment of peripheral circulation disorders. *Helv Chir Acta.* 1954;21(5–6):499.

Fox KA, Dabbous OH, Goldberg RJ, et al. Prediction of risk of death and myocardial infarction in the six months after presentation with acute coronary syndrome: prospective multinational observational study (GRACE). *BMJ.* 2006; 333(7578):1091.

Friberg L, Rosenqvist M, Lip GY. Evaluation of risk stratification schemes for ischaemic stroke and bleeding in 182 678 patients with atrial fibrillation: the Swedish Atrial Fibrillation cohort study. *Eur Heart J.* 2012;33:1500.

Galie N, Sais F, Palazzini M, et al. Left main coronary artery compression in patients with pulmonary arterial hypertension and angina. *JACC.* 2017;69:2808–2817.

Goff DC Jr, Lloyd-Jones DM, Bennett G, et al. 2013 ACC/AHA guideline on the assessment of cardiovascular risk: a report of the American College of Cardiology/American Heart Association Task Force on Practice Guidelines. *Circulation.* 2014;129(25)(suppl 2):S49.

Grossman W. *Profiles in Valvular Heart Disease. Grossman's Cardiac Catheterization, Angiography and Intervention.* Edited by Baim D, Grossman W. Philadelphia, PA: Lippincott Williams & Wilkins; 2000: 759–84. 6

Hochman JS, Sleeper LA, Webb JG, et al. Effect of early revascularization for cardiogenic shock on 1-year mortality: the SHOCK Trial results. *Circulation.* 1999;100:I–369.

Hunt SA, Abraham WT, Chin MH, et al. ACC/AHA 2005 guideline update for the diagnosis and management of chronic heart failure in the adult. *Circulation.* 2005;112 (12): e154–235.

James PA, Oparil S, Carter BL, et al. 2014 evidence-based guideline for the management of high blood pressure in adults: report from the panel members appointed to the Eighth Joint National Committee (JNC 8). *JAMA.* 2014;311(5):507.

January CT, Wann LS, Alpert JS, et al. 2014 AHA/ACC/HRS guideline for the management of patients with atrial fibrillation: a report of the American College of Cardiology/American Heart Association Task Force on Practice Guidelines and the Heart Rhythm Society. *J Am Coll Cardiol.* 2014; 130(23):2071–2104.

Killip T III, Kimball JT. Treatment of myocardial infarction in a coronary care unit: a two year experience with 250 patients. *Am J Cardiol.* 1967;20(4):457.

Krone RJ, Laskey WK, Johnson C, et al. A simplified lesion classification for predicting success and complications of coronary angioplasty. *Am J Cardiol.* 2000;85:1179–1184.

Li JS, Sexton DJ, Mick N, et al. Proposed modifications to the Duke Criteria for the diagnosis of infective endocarditis. *Clinical Infectious Diseases.* 2000; 30(4): 633–638.

Lip GY. Implications of the CHA2DS2-VASc and HAS-BLED scores for thromboprophylaxis in atrial fibrillation. *Am J Med.* 2011;124:111.

Mann DL, Zipes DP, Libby P, et al. *Braunwald's Heart Disease: A Textbook of Cardiovascular Medicine.* 10th ed. Philadelphia, PA: Elsevier/Saunders; 2015.

Mark DB, Hlatky MA, Harrell FE Jr, et al. Exercise treadmill score for predicting prognosis in coronary artery disease. *Ann Intern Med.* 1987;106(6):793.

McMurray JJV, Packer M, Desai AS, et al for the PARADIGM-HF Investigators and Committees. Angiotensin–Neprilysin Inhibition versus Enalapril in heart failure. *N Engl J Med.* 2014; 371:993–1004.

Mehran R, Aymong ED, Nikolsky E, et al. A simple risk score for prediction of contrast-induced nephropathy after percutaneous coronary intervention: development and initial validation. *J Am Coll Cardiol.* 2004; 44(7):1393–1399.

Mehran R, Rao SV, Bhatt DL, et al. Standardized bleeding definitions for cardiovascular clinical trials: a consensus report from the Bleeding Academic Research Consortium. *Circulation.* 2011;123:2736.

Morrow DA, Antman EM, Charlesworth A, et al. TIMI risk score for ST-elevation myocardial infarction: a convenient, bedside, clinical score for risk assessment at presentation: an intravenous nPA for treatment of infarcting myocardium early II trial substudy. *Circulation.* 2000;102(17):2031–2037.

Murphy JG, Lloyd MA, eds. *Mayo Clinic Cardiology: Concise Textbook.* 4th ed. New York: Mayo Clinic Scientific Press/ Oxford University Press; 2013.

Norgren L, Hiatt WR, Dormandy JA, et al. Inter-Society Consensus for the Management of Peripheral Arterial Disease (TASC II). *J Vasc Surg.* 2007;45(suppl S):S5.

Otto C. *Valvular Heart Disease.* Philadelphia, PA: Saunders Elsevier;2004: 404–405.

Ridker PM, Buring JE, Rifai N, et al. Development and validation of improved algorithms for the assessment of global cardiovascular risk in women: the Reynolds Risk Score. *JAMA.* 2007;297(6):611.

Rogers JH, Lasala JM. Coronary artery dissection and perforation complicating percutaneous coronary intervention. *J Invasive Cardiol.* 2004;16(9):493–499.

Rutherford RB, Baker JD, Ernst C, et al. Recommended standards for reports dealing with lower extremity ischemia: revised version. *J Vasc Surg.* 1997;26(3):517.

Ryan TJ, Faxon DP, Gunnar RM, et al. Guidelines for percutaneous transluminal coronary angioplasty. A report of the American College of Cardiology/American Heart Association Task Force on Assessment of Diagnostic and Therapeutic Cardiovascular Procedures (Subcommittee on Percutaneous Transluminal Coronary Angioplasty). *Circulation.* 1988;78:486–502.

Serruys PW, Morice MC, Kappetein AP, et al. Percutaneous coronary intervention versus coronary-artery bypass grafting for severe coronary artery disease. *N Engl J Med.* 2009; 360(10):961.

SHOCK Investigators, Hochman JS, Sleeper LA, et al. Early revascularization in acute myocardial infarction complicated by cardiogenic shock. *N Engl J Med.* 1999;341: 625–634.

Simonneau G, Robbins I, Beghetti M, et al. Updated clinical classification of pulmonary hypertension. *J Am Coll Cardiol.* 2009;54:S43–S54.

Smith SW, Dodd KW, Henry TD, et al. Diagnosis of ST-elevation myocardial infarction in the presence of left bundle branch block with the ST-elevation to S-wave ratio in a modified Sgarbossa rule. *Ann Emerg Med.* 2012;60(6):766–776.

The Criteria Committee of the New York Heart Association. *Nomenclature and Criteria for Diagnosis of Diseases of the Heart and Great Vessels.* 9th ed. Boston: Little, Brown & Co.; 1994: 253–256.

Thygesen K, Alpert JS, Jaffe AS, et al. (24 August 2012). Third universal definition of myocardial infarction. *Circulation.* 2012;126(16): 2020–2035.

Wilson PW, D'Agostino RB, Levy D, et al. Prediction of coronary heart disease using risk factor categories. *Circulation.* 1998;97(18):1837–1847.

Index

About the Author

DR. YEREM YEGHIAZARIANS is the Leone-Perkins Family Endowed Chair in Cardiology and professor of medicine at University of California, San Francisco (UCSF). He serves as Director of the Translational Cardiac Stem Cell Program, Co-Director of the Adult Cardiac Catheterization Laboratory and Director of the Peripheral Interventional Cardiology Program, and previously served as the President of the San Francisco Board of the American Heart Association from 2013–2016. He has received numerous teaching awards and he is very active in the education of medical students, internal medicine residents, and cardiology fellows at UCSF.

Dr. Yeghiazarians received his undergraduate degree in Biology/Biochemistry from Brandeis University (1991) and his medical degree from The Johns Hopkins School of Medicine (1995). He trained in internal medicine, general and interventional cardiology at The Brigham and Women's Hospital, Harvard Medical School, where he also served as chief medical resident prior to joining UCSF in 2003. He has a broad background in general cardiology, interventional cardiology and clinical/basic research, and has authored over 100 manuscripts and book chapters. He is also co-editor of *Handbook of Endovascular Peripheral Interventions*.

CPSIA information can be obtained
at www.ICGtesting.com
Printed in the USA
LVOW13s0918261217
560762LV00002B/2/P

9 780813 579689